Lavender

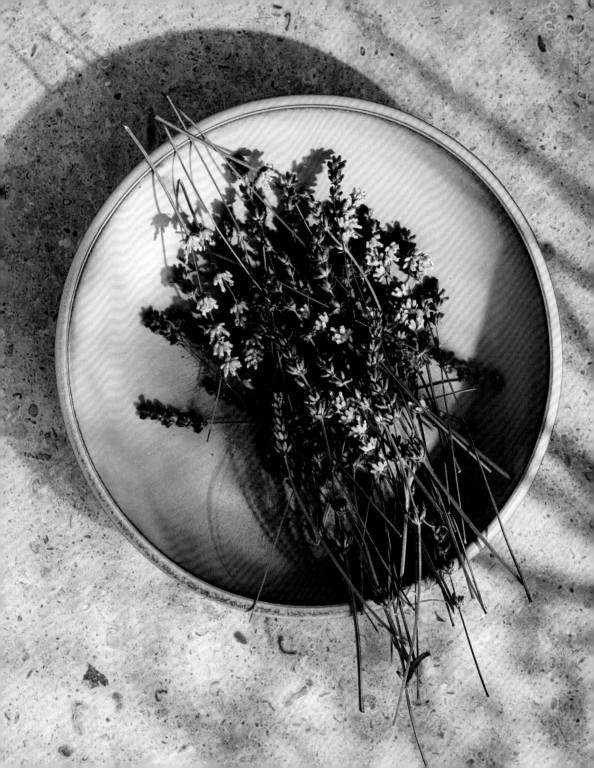

Lavender

50 SELF-CARE RECIPES AND PROJECTS FOR NATURAL WELLNESS

Bonnie Louise Gillis

Photography by Charity Burggraaf

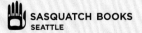

SASQUATCH BOOKS
SEATTLE

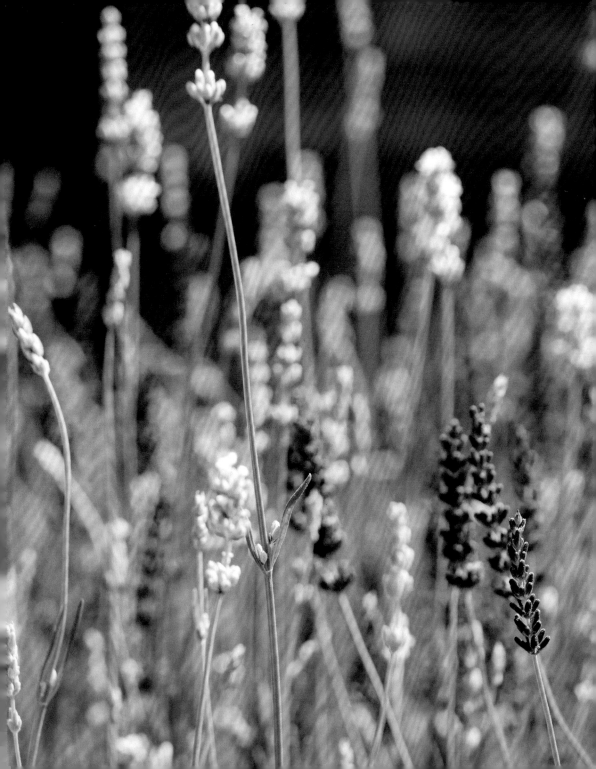

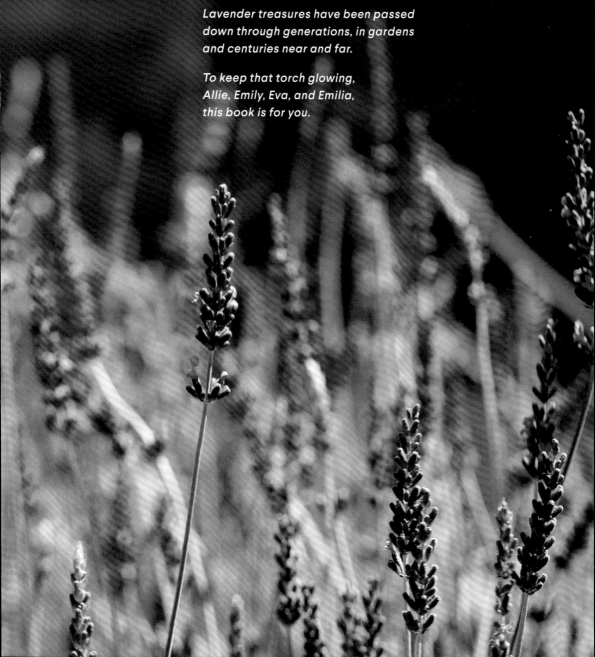

Lavender treasures have been passed
down through generations, in gardens
and centuries near and far.

To keep that torch glowing,
Allie, Emily, Eva, and Emilia,
this book is for you.

Contents

130 TASTE

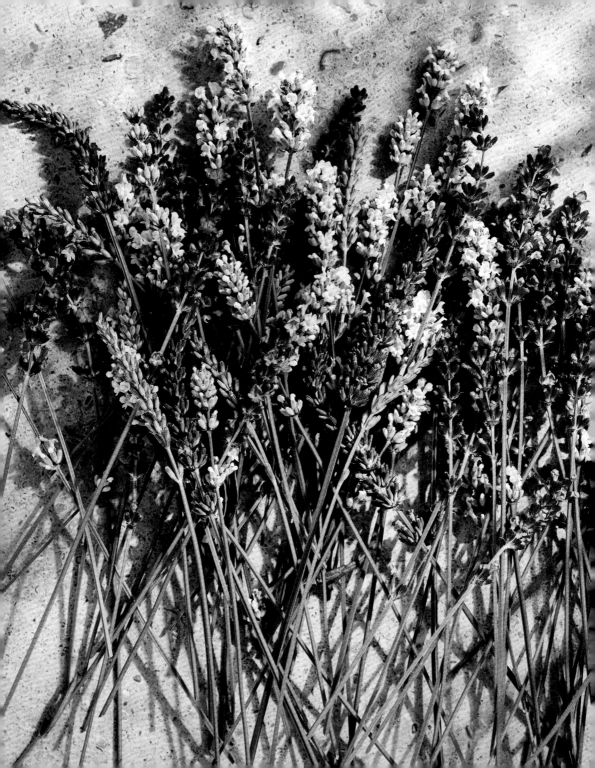

Introduction

Lavender has wafted its way around the world and through the pages of recorded history. Like an amulet, the herb was dangled to chase away demons, moths, and disease, and its oil was prescribed for headaches, hysteria, and gas. When Europe was ravaged by plagues, lavender was stuffed into the beaks of bird-shaped masks to ward off the Black Death—a disease that people thought was transmitted by scent.

Hidden within many myths are buds of truth, and so it is with lavender. The clean, powerful scent of the herb did indeed protect some from plagues as it fragranced the air, but not because it banished the evil smell of disease. Science has shown that those diseases were often carried by fleas on rats, and the scent of lavender repelled both rodents and biting insects. Thanks to modern science we also know that lavender essential oil does indeed contain some disinfecting, soothing, relaxing, and pain-relieving properties.

Lavender continues to scent our modern world, appearing in culinary seasonings, household cleaners, and aromatherapy. But with one significant change. Lavender's resurgence is now fueled by science instead of superstition, and by delight instead of desperation.

Read on, and you'll discover numerous practical ways you can harness the calming and healing properties of lavender in your garden, home, kitchen, body, mind, and life. This timeless herb has truly earned its place in today's society as a potent and delectable ingredient for wellness.

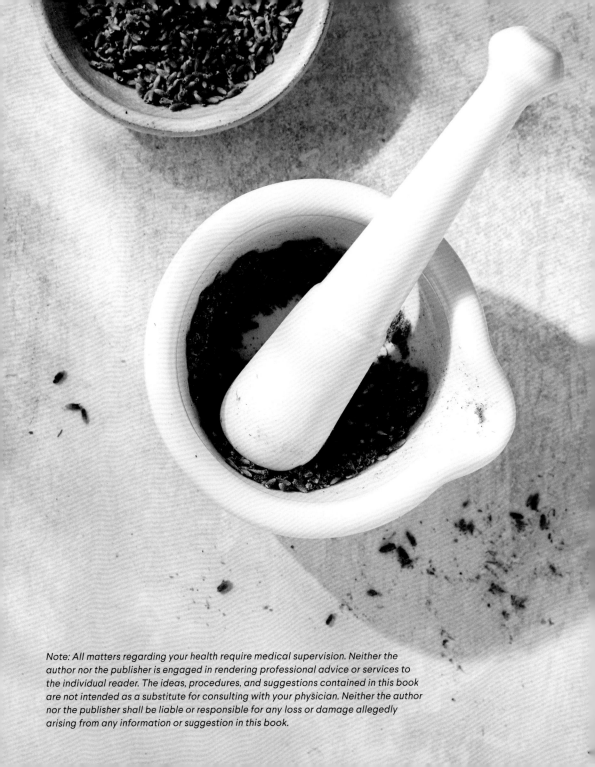

Safety

Natural is sometimes confused with *safe*. But even poison hemlock is natural, and so are tornadoes. Like any powerful natural element, essential oils and herbs carry risks. Be sure to read and understand the following considerations before exploring the natural recipes in this book.

PRECAUTIONS

THERAPEUTIC USE. Before using any essential oil, consult your primary care physician. The essential oil blends included here were tested by an aromatherapist with decades of professional experience. However, the blends and recipes are merely suggestions for complementary therapy and are not a substitute for professional medical care or prescriptions. Lavender essential oil is not effective against viruses, including coronaviruses like COVID-19.

SIDE EFFECTS. If you experience a reaction that is serious or systemic, seek medical help. Most adverse reactions are linked with essential oil oxidation, adulteration, substitution, or toxic dosing. Other side effects have resulted from allergies, drug interactions, or comorbidities.

DROWSINESS. The relaxing effects of *L. angustifolia* may cause drowsiness. If you experience a sedative reaction to lavender, do not drive or operate machinery during use.

SENSITIZATION. Overuse of any natural product can lead to sensitization to its chemical components. For best results and longevity of use, rotate the essential oils and cleaning products you use and apply them sparingly. Linalool is a primary component of lavender that has been added to a multitude of skin-care products from facial creams to foot peels. Hundreds of commercial household products contain linalool as well. Sensitization to linalool has caused hives or dermatitis in some users.

BLENDS. Before blending any oils with lavender, research the warnings, drug interactions, possible reactions, and contra-indications for those oils.

PURCHASING

PURITY. Essential oil quality and purity are not regulated by any government agency. Many oils from unscrupulous sellers have been adulterated with synthetics or cheaper oils to increase profit or lower prices. If you purchase oil for culinary use or for its therapeutic qualities, buy only 100 percent pure essential oil from a source that has earned your full confidence. Avoid oil made from lavender that may have been grown with pesticides, including lavender intended for crafts or décor.

SPECIES. For most lavender aromatherapy and culinary use, the label should state *L. angustifolia* and no other ingredients. If your purpose allows or requires higher camphor content, the label may state *L. x intermedia* or lavandin. Avoid essential oil made from other lavender species unless directed by a professional.

PACKAGING. Chemical compounds in essential oils lose their effectiveness and become allergenic or contaminated if the oil is packaged improperly. See How to Store Lavender Oil on page 55.

USES

TOPICAL. Do not apply essential oil to any open wound with deep broken layers of skin or tissue without your doctor's recommendation. Patch test any essential oil before applying it to your skin. If redness or irritation appears, stop using and wash the area with gentle soap and warm water. Do not attempt to alleviate irritation with another essential oil. Avoid mucous membranes, such as nasal passages, lips, mouth, vagina, or anus. Wash hands with soap and warm water after working with or applying essential oils to avoid accidentally rubbing eyes or other sensitive areas. Never put undiluted essential oil in or near eyes. If essential oil splashes into your eye, immediately flush the eye under running water for 15 minutes. Seek medical help if irritation continues.

DIFFUSER. Diffuser recipes are not safe for topical use. When diffusing essential oils, if you feel any airway irritation, discontinue use and get some fresh air. If you experience any breathing difficulty, seek medical help.

Patch Test for Reactions

Apply 1 undiluted drop of lavender essential oil to a clean, dry area of soft skin, such as the crook of your elbow. Cover with a waterproof bandage. Wait 48 hours, monitoring for skin reactions such as redness, swelling, or itching. Some doctors recommend waiting a week. If you notice irritation, remove the bandage, wash with soap and water, and avoid using that oil. Note that a patch test does not prevent future sensitization to an oil, which commonly results from overexposure to any natural component.

Note: Some other essential oils are considered *hot* oils (such as oregano, thyme, and clove) and need to be diluted prior to patch testing.

ORAL. Don't ingest essential oil unless directed by a doctor who knows your full medical history and current prescriptions. Lavender essential oil is "Generally Recognized As Safe" (GRAS) by the Food and Drug Administration (FDA) *only* as a flavoring, such as 1 or 2 drops added to food. The FDA has not approved lavender oil for medicinal purposes.[1] Before drinking herbal tea, consult with a doctor if you are nursing, pregnant, taking medications, or scheduled for surgery. Avoid making tea from any plant to which you are allergic.

BATHTUB. When adding oil of any kind to a bath, use extra caution to prevent slipping in the tub. If you experience irritation, discontinue use and wash with gentle soap and warm water. If you are pregnant, or have diabetes, wounds, infections, blood pressure issues, or compromised health, check with your doctor before taking a hot bath.

STEAM. Hot steam can burn skin and tissue. Approach steam slowly and cautiously. Avoid steam inhalation if you have asthma.[2] Heated steam can also aggravate rosacea and inflammatory acne symptoms.

SPRAY. When spraying the air with essential oils, avoid contact with eyes, and do not spray near children.

RESTRICTIONS

SURGERY. Stop using lavender oil 2 weeks prior to surgery to prevent possible interactions with anesthesia and other surgery-related medications.

EPILEPSY. If you are at risk of seizures, don't use any essential oils without your doctor's approval.

HEART CONDITIONS. Essential oils that contain stimulating chemicals, including high-camphor lavender, can increase blood pressure.

ESTROGEN-DEPENDENT CANCER. Avoid lavender oil if you have this form of cancer.

PREGNANCY AND BREASTFEEDING. Not enough is known about possible effects of lavender oil on unborn or nursing babies. If you are pregnant or breastfeeding, do not use any essential oils unless approved by your doctor.

CHILDREN. Keep essential oils secured and out of reach of young hands. The effects of lavender essential oil for those under the age of puberty are debated and undetermined. Due to possible hormone disruption, usage is not recommended unless specifically approved by your child's physician.

ELDERLY OR IMMUNOCOMPROMISED ADULTS. Don't expose anyone to aromatherapy whose health is compromised unless usage is approved by their physician, and then use no more than half the drops of essential oil recommended for a healthy adult.

PETS. Before using essential oils in a pet environment, consult your veterinarian. Lavender essential oil is *not* safe for use with birds or most small animals. A diffuser should never be used if birds are present. Misuse of lavender oil can also be dangerous with cats.

Always be mindful of your pet's acute sense of smell. Make sure your pet can leave the scented area at will. Lavender is often used to calm nerves and skin irritation in dogs, but reports of lavender essential oil misuse with dogs are linked to upset tummies, skin rashes, and emotional distress. According to veterinarian Dr. Michael T. Nappier, "Dogs have up to 300 million olfactory receptors in their noses, versus only about 6 million for us. And the part of their brain dedicated to inter-preting these is about 40 times larger than ours. A dog's sense of smell can detect the equivalent of ½ teaspoon of sugar in an Olympic-sized swimming pool."[3]

Grow

It's natural to breathe a little deeper once you've entered a garden, especially when the fragrance of lavender floats through the air. Numerous studies show that horticultural therapy, which is a kind of rehabilitation that includes walking or working in a garden, lowers blood pressure, pulse rate, and the stress hormone cortisol.

Urban environments can trigger stress. They overload the senses and keep your defenses high. While antioxidant-rich foods and aromatherapy help to remedy the harmful effects of chronic stress on the body, horticultural therapy actually lowers stress itself.

Growing lavender offers rewards that far outweigh the labor to grow it, even if your garden is simply a collection of pots on a balcony or in a sunny window. Just a couple of lavender plants can supply you with enough organic flowers for all your cooking and home-fragrance needs.

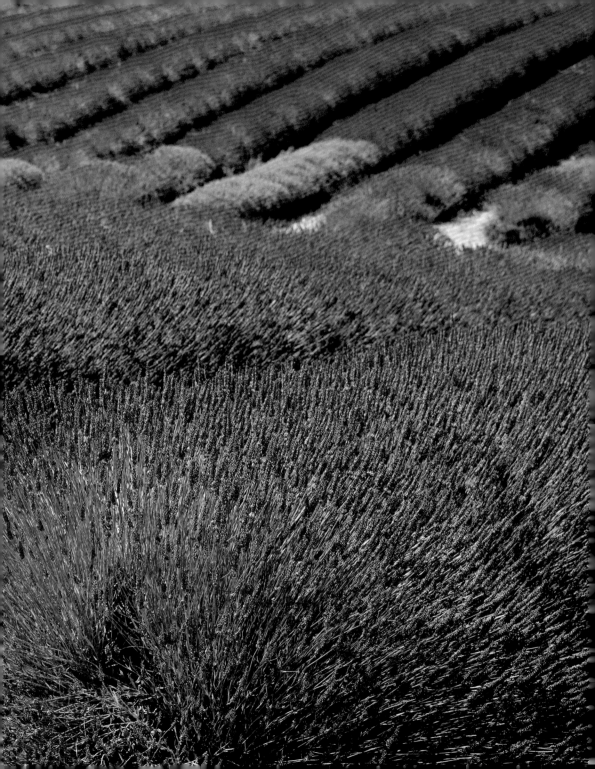

THE MANY FACES & NAMES OF LAVENDER

At least 45 distinct species of lavender grow around the world. All of them belong to the genus *Lavandula* (*L.*). Within those species, more than 450 unique varieties and cultivars of lavender have been named. Most lavenders sold today are cultivars, but the word *cultivar*, which means a plant variety that's been selected and cultivated by humans, is rarely used by retailers, so for simplicity you'll see *variety* here for both natural and cultivated lavenders.

The most common species of lavender have multiple nicknames, depending on where you live or who is talking. For instance "French lavender" is the common nickname for three entirely different species. The clearest way to identify a lavender species is by its Latin name, so that's what you'll see in this book. One exception is the popular hybrid species *L. x intermedia*. It is commonly called "lavandin" without confusion, so for simplicity you'll see lavandin used here.

Abbreviations

L.	*Lavandula* (genus of lavender)
lavandin	*L. x intermedia* (most common hybrid species)
lavender oil	Lavender essential oil
variety	Cultivar or variety of lavender

COMMON LAVENDER SPECIES

All species of lavender belong to the mint family (Lamiaceae), each one set apart by differences among leaves, flowers, aromas, and essential oils. On the following pages are four of the most commonly grown species of lavender.

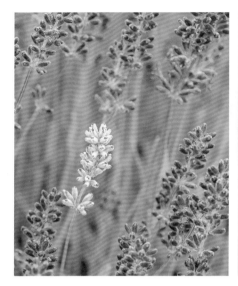 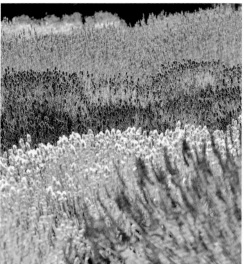

CLIMATE: Hardy in zones 5 to 9; requires low humidity

BLOOM TIME: Typically between May and July, depending on climate

SCENT: Sweet and floral

CHEMICAL PROPERTIES: Soothing and relaxing

Lavandula angustifolia

Dubbed with names such as "common," "true," or "English" lavender, this is the most cold-hardy species. The sweetest perfumes and deepest blues also come from *L. angustifolia*, along with soft pastels, such as white, pink, periwinkle, and classic lavender. The essential oil has a delicate fragrance and is highly sought after for aromatherapy, fine perfumes, and culinary uses.

You might expect—given its desirability and higher cost—that you would prefer the scent of *L. angustifolia*. And you might. But the fragrance most associated with lavender comes from lavandin. Don't be surprised if you find yourself drawn to the more affordable, more familiar scent.

When *L. angustifolia* plants are grown from seed, cross-pollination creates variations that aren't true to type. If you want a specific variety of *L. angustifolia*, choose plants grown from cuttings ("clonal" lavender), or you could be disappointed with the plant's bloom color and full-grown size.

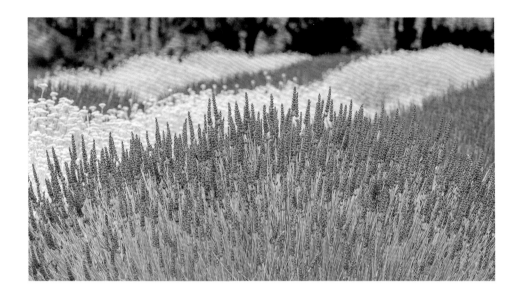

CLIMATE: Hardy in zones 5 to 9; tolerates some humidity

BLOOM TIME: Usually a few weeks later than *L. angustifolia*

SCENT: Sharply fragrant

CHEMICAL PROPERTIES: Either invigorating and penetrating, or calming, depending on variety

Lavandula x *intermedia* (lavandin)

Lavandin is the labradoodle of the lavender world. From one lavender parent comes winterhardiness and a sweet scent. From the other, longer stems, a higher yield of oil, and a sharper camphor scent (think muscle-rubs).

This hybrid first appeared when bees cross-pollinated two species in neighboring fields. As a mule, it can only be reproduced from cuttings, but the flowers are rich with nectar. Its blooms arrive while *L. angustifolia*'s color is fading, so by layering both species into your garden, you can stretch your viewing pleasure and fill your garden with happy bees.

Note: You can find your climate zone on the USDA Plant Hardiness Zone Map, which is displayed at PlantHardiness.ars.usda.gov/PHZMWeb.

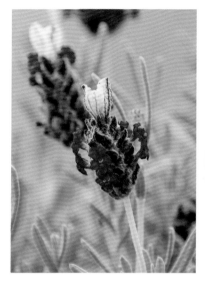
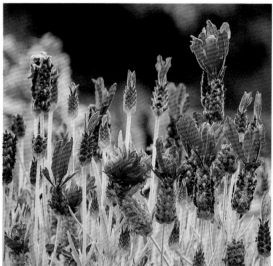

CLIMATE: Hardy in zones 8 to 9; tolerates humidity

BLOOM TIME: Continuously from spring to frost; needs regular trimming

SCENT: Pungent and minty

CHEMICAL PROPERTIES: Antimicrobial

Lavandula stoechas

Known for nonstop blooming and distinctive bracts atop their pineapple-shaped heads, *L. stoechas* has earned such nicknames as "rabbit ears" and "butterfly" lavender. Outstanding colors include whites, yellows, violets, and some of the brightest pinks of all lavenders.

Popular in southern regions, this species typically thrives in tropical climates. In northern climes, varieties are grown as annuals or confined to pots. *Lavandula stoechas* is a highly prolific seeder that was branded an invasive weed in parts of Australia.

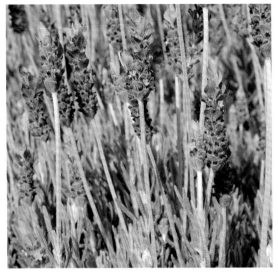 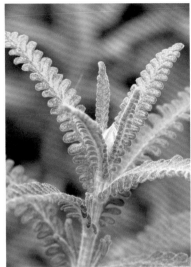

CLIMATE: Hardy in zones 8 to 10; tolerates humidity

BLOOM TIME: Continuously from spring to frost; needs regular trimming

SCENT: Floral-eucalyptus

CHEMICAL PROPERTIES: Antibacterial and insect-repelling

Lavandula dentata

Aptly called "toothed" or "fringed" lavender for the scalloped edging around each little leaf, *L. dentata* is a tender plant best suited for deserts and tropics. Native to areas surrounding the Middle East, the species can be found thriving in places like California, Texas, Florida, Africa, and Australia.

Lavandula dentata can be potted and carried to warm shelter in colder climates, where its unique foliage may be evergreen.

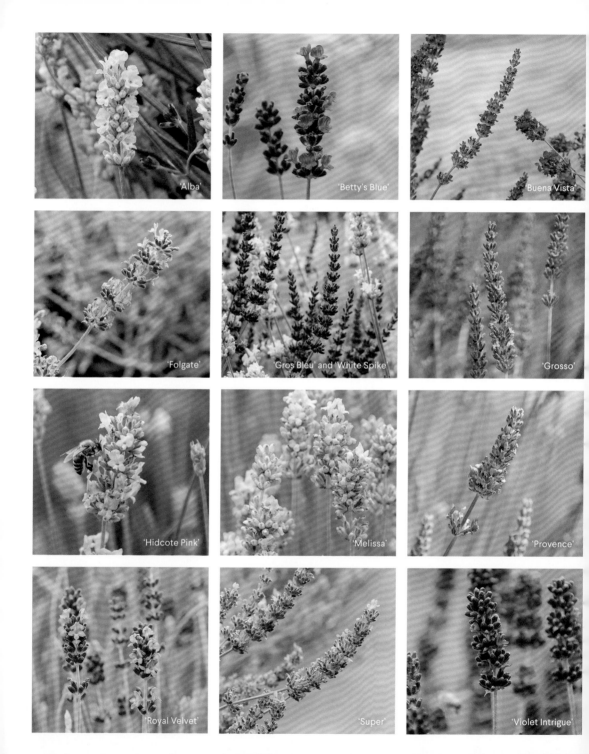

'Alba'

'Betty's Blue'

'Buena Vista'

'Folgate'

'Gros Bleu' and 'White Spike'

'Grosso'

'Hidcote Pink'

'Melissa'

'Provence'

'Royal Velvet'

'Super'

'Violet Intrigue'

FAVORITE GARDEN VARIETIES

Climate dictates which species are able to flourish in your region, but you can choose from many exceptional varieties. If your area is especially cold, hot, or humid, visit a locally owned nursery or lavender farm to see which varieties are thriving there. Consider these choices when shopping for lavender plants:

PLANT SIZE. Choose from dwarf, standard, or large.

FRAGRANCE. Scent may be sweet, sharp, or pungent.

BLOOM COLOR. Select from a spectrum of pastel and vibrant shades.

FOLIAGE. Leaves range from green to silvery gray, from smooth to fuzzy, and from narrow to scalloped.

LENGTH OF FLOWER STEMS. Stem length varies from 4 inches to more than 2 feet.

SIZE OF FLOWER HEAD. Choose short, plump, long, or slender.

Pacific Northwest Favorites

Temperate climates with wet winters and dry summers:

Lavandula angustifolia
'Alba'
'Betty's Blue'
'Buena Vista'
'Folgate'
'Hidcote Pink'
'Melissa'
'Royal Velvet'
'Violet Intrigue'

Lavandula x intermedia
'Fred Boutin'
'Gros Bleu'
'Grosso'
'Provence'
'Super'
'White Spike'

Midwest Favorites	Cold, windy winters such as those in the Midwest plains, Colorado, and Ontario:	
	Lavandula angustifolia 'Betty's Blue' 'Croxton's Wild' 'Folgate' 'Imperial Gem'	'Munstead' 'Royal Velvet' *Lavandula x intermedia* 'Phenomenal'

Northeast Favorites	Cold, blustery winters and humid summers:	
	Lavandula angustifolia 'Hidcote' 'Munstead'	*Lavandula x intermedia* 'Phenomenal' 'Provence'

Deep South Favorites	An abundance of heat and humidity:	
	Lavandula angustifolia Not recommended for humid climates

Lavandula x intermedia 'Phenomenal' 'Provence'

Lavandula dentata All varieties; often sold as "French" or "fern-leaf" lavender (look for toothed leaves) | *Lavandula stoechas (pedunculata)* Often sold as "Spanish lavender" (look for bunny ears atop flowers) 'Ballerina' 'Bandera Pink' 'Kew Red' 'Lemon Leigh' 'Otto Quast' 'White Anouk' |

Southwest Desert Favorites

Dry air and scorching summer heat:

Lavandula angustifolia
'Hidcote'
'Munstead'
'Royal Velvet'

Lavandula x *intermedia*
'Grosso'

Lavandula dentata
All varieties; often sold as "French" or "fern-leaf" lavender (look for toothed leaves)

Lavandula stoechas (pedunculata)
All varieties; often sold as "Spanish lavender" (look for bunny ears atop flowers)

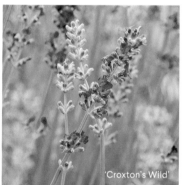
'Croxton's Wild'

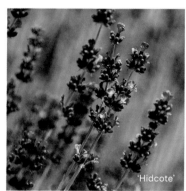
'Hidcote'

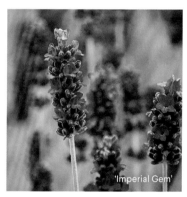
'Imperial Gem'

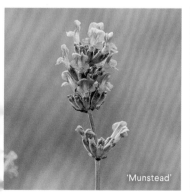
'Munstead'

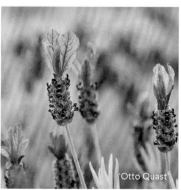
'Otto Quast'

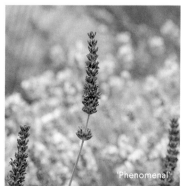
'Phenomenal'

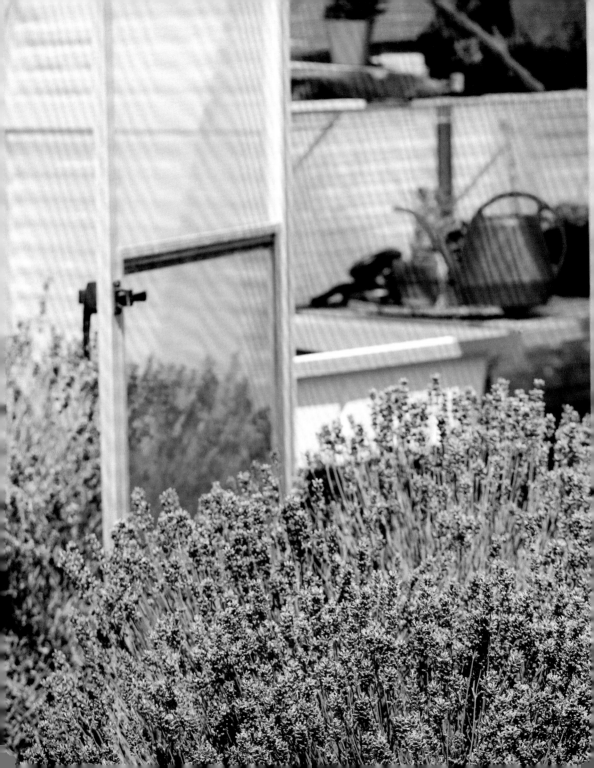

HOW TO GROW LAVENDER

The more closely you can mimic lavender's native home, the happier your plant will be. The origins of early lavender trace to cliffs of the Mediterranean, where millennia of winds and storms swept the highland soil into the valleys below, leaving behind rocky cliffs with meager, stubborn dirt that is rich in limestone and low in nitrogen.

Soil Can Kill

Waterlogged soil is the most common reason lavender plants fail. Lavender likes dry feet. It needs water to run quickly from its 12-inch-deep roots. A sandy loam and porous, rocky soil suit lavender well, and so does an elevated bed.

Root rot—most commonly *Phytophthora*—is a disease that thrives in slow-draining, dense soil. It will kill your lavender. If your soil is a heavy clay or caliche, plant on a hillside or berm, or in a mound or porous container. As needed, fluff up your soil with grit, pea gravel, and sand to create a quick-draining bed that is at least ⅓ inorganic filler.

The pH Sweet Spot

Ranging from acidic to alkaline, the pH level of your soil is important. Lavender cannot get the nutrients it needs from a low pH (acidic) soil. It prefers a pH near 7. Check your soil with a pH tester, and amend it with garden lime if needed to raise the pH level to at least 6.5, but not higher than 7.5.

Planting

Dig a hole 18 inches deep and 12 inches wider than the roots of your plant. Toss in a layer of rocks, a layer of coarse compost, and then some amended (fluffy, rocky, quick-draining) soil mix. Place the lavender into the hole so that the crown (where roots meet stem) sits slightly above the surface. Fill the hole with soil mix so the crown is barely covered. Compact the soil lightly around the plant and water thoroughly.

Tips for Healthy Lavender Plants

Healthy lavender is tough, resilient, and rarely infected or infested. But for all its superpowers, a puddle of water is lavender's kryptonite. Nearly every lavender casualty can be avoided with a few precautions:

FOSTER STRONG ROOTS. Avoid conditions that weaken roots, such as overwatering, dense soil, poor drainage, insufficient sunlight, and acidic soil.

ALLOW AIR TO FLOW. Leave space between plants. Prune at least once a year. Avoid landscape fabric.

WATER ONLY THE ROOTS. Avoid overhead watering.

PRACTICE GOOD GARDEN HYGIENE. Sanitize pruners before and after trimming each plant to help prevent disease. Soaking and dipping tools in full-strength household cleaners such as Lysol and Pine-Sol are recommended. Wiping blades with rubbing alcohol can be effective too.[1] Avoid contaminated soil, and sanitize pots if you reuse them.

REMOVE NESTING ATTRACTIONS FOR INSECTS AND RODENTS. Keep birdseed away from the garden. Trim or remove dense ground-level vegetation. Pull weeds. Rake out leaf litter and winter debris. Remove thick mulch that is close to shrubs and trees.

ATTRACT BENEFICIAL PREDATORS. Increase ladybugs, lacewings, dragonflies, hummingbirds, and spiders by planting a diversity of plants. Do not use pesticides.

SHELTER LAVENDER FROM ICE AND ICY WINDS. Consider planting a windbreak or constructing a stone wall if needed. Cover plants with light fabric as needed in winter to prevent ice from coating the branches.

REMEDY DISEASES AND BLIGHTS. Susceptibility varies by region, climate, soil, and species of lavender. Some problems are tough to diagnose, some are contagious, and most are diffi-cult to remedy organically. Seek help from a nursery, county extension office, or horticulturist in your area.

Spacing

It's tempting to fill all the empty space in a garden, but to help prevent harmful fungi, give lavender enough space for air to circulate around its foliage. Plan for lavender to double in size every year for the first 3 years. Space average-sized lavender plants about 3 feet apart.

Fertilizing

Lavender fares poorly in rich soil and can't survive salty manure or nitrogen-based fertilizers for long. Test your soil in the spring, and if needed, feed once with an organic, slow-release fertilizer. The type of fertilizer you choose will depend on the needs of your soil. If the soil is too acidic, scratch some lime into the soil to adjust the pH level. If your soil lacks phosphorous, add some bonemeal in the fall. Prolific bloomers such as *L. stoechas* and *L. dentata* may prefer a monthly feeding when in bloom.

Topdressing

Topdressing depends on your climate:

HOT, ARID CLIMATES. Natural bark mulch helps the soil retain moisture. Keep mulch 2 to 3 inches away from the crown.

COOL, WET, AND/OR HUMID CLIMATES. Light-colored gravel or pebbles, white sand, or crushed oyster-shell mulch can help drainage, reflect heat back up to foliage, and prevent patho-genic soil from splashing onto the leaves.

Sunlight

Whether in-ground or indoors, lavender needs at least 6 hours of full sun daily, all year round. Indoors, natural light can be supplemented with LED grow lights if needed.

Water

Overhead watering creates a damp breeding ground for leaf fungi, so try to water the lavender roots instead of foliage. If that's not possible, water early in the morning to allow leaves plenty of time to dry before temperatures drop in the evening.

FIRST-YEAR PLANTS. After planting, soak thoroughly and count the days until the leaves begin to slightly close up to conserve moisture. Then soak again. This will give you a feel for how many days to allow between regular soakings. Count days again at the beginning of each new weather season.

ESTABLISHED ROOTS. Soil that is dry from lack of spring rain needs a good soaking when plants begin to bud. Although drought tolerant, lavender roots may need some watering during hot, dry seasons. Frequency will depend on your climate and soil. Let soil dry out between waterings, watch for signs of stress, and then give roots a deep soaking. Some growers recommend a deep soaking right after harvest.

Pruning

A compact mound of lavender is less vulnerable to winter damage than leggy branches. Prune at summer's end if you don't harvest your lavender flowers, or if your plants have a second flush of blooms after harvesting, or if you don't shape your lavender at the time you harvest. Pruning also increases the vigor and life span of the plant. Without regular trimming, more and more of the lavender plant will become woody, weak, and unproductive over time.

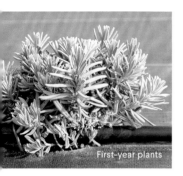

First-year plants

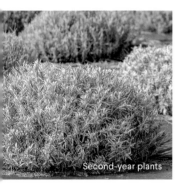

Second-year plants

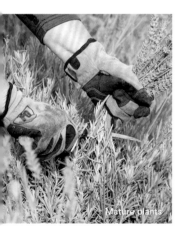

Mature plants

Lavandula angustifolia & lavandin

FIRST-YEAR PLANTS. Thick, bare wood at the base of the plant has no nodes from which to send out new shoots, so you need to leave some leafy softwood stem intact. Grasp the handful of stalks and use hand pruners to cut through stems a couple of inches above the leafless wood. Lavender farmers recommend doing this every week during the plant's first growing season. You will sacrifice first-year blooms but gain a larger, fuller plant in the coming year.

SECOND-YEAR PLANTS. With hand pruners, cut through stems a couple of inches above the bare wood, leaving a few nodes on each branch. Trim around the edges of the plant as needed to shape into a compact mound.

MATURE PLANTS. After the third year, your plant will be fully grown. Depending on the variety of lavender, your trimmed mound may be 1 to 3 feet in diameter. With mature plants, working with a harvesting scythe (a serrated sickle) is easier and will allow you to prune an entire plant in about 10 minutes. As in previous years, leave a couple of inches of nodes above each bare-wood branch.

Lavandula stoechas & Lavandula dentata

Fully prune tender tropicals after their brilliant spring show. With hand pruners, remove blooms plus about ⅓ of the leafy part of the stem. Shape plant into a rounded mound. Because they bloom continuously, you'll be forced to sacrifice emerging blooms when you remove the faded spring flush. Chopping off lovely buds is painful for any gardener, but you'll be rewarded with plenty of fresh blooms during the summer, and then fuller lavender plants the following spring.

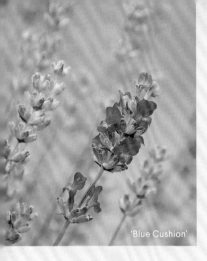

'Blue Cushion'

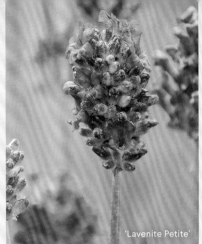

'Lavenite Petite'

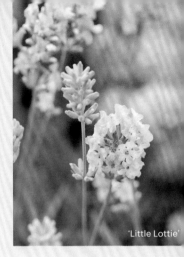

'Little Lottie'

Growing Lavender in Containers

Although lavender prefers an in-ground, outdoor bed, many varieties adapt well to pot life when their needs are met.

TEMPERATURE. During the summer, container soil may be 20 degrees hotter than in-ground soil. Daytime temperatures in excess of 90 degrees can quickly kill potted lavender roots. When temperatures dip into the mid-40s, container soil may be 15 degrees colder, which can also kill lavender roots that are not winter-hardy.

POT SIZE. A small pot is fine for first-year lavender, but in the spring you'll need to transplant to a larger pot that is 16 to 24 inches wide with several ½-inch drainage holes. In extreme temperature climates, your pot needs to be at least 2 feet wide to allow for soil insulation around the roots.

OXYGEN. Choose containers made from porous materials that can breathe, such as terra-cotta pots.

SOIL. Begin with a layer of rocks at the bottom. Add some quick-draining potting soil mixed with nonorganic filler, such as pea gravel or garden sand, at a ratio of ⅔ soil to ⅓ filler. Many potted-soil mixes are too acidic for lavender, so amend with lime if needed to raise pH, ideally between 6.5 and 7.0.

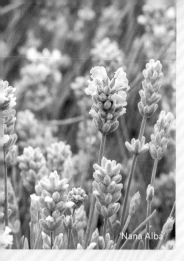

'Nana Alba'

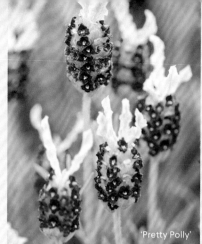

'Pretty Polly'

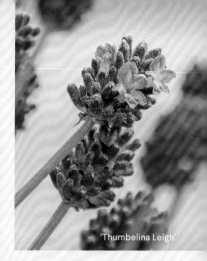

'Thumbelina Leigh'

SUNLIGHT. Inside or out, lavender needs at least 6 hours a day of sunlight.

WATER. Drench roots with water when soil feels dry a few inches below the surface.

DWARF VARIETIES. The shrubby base of some lavenders grow 3 feet wide and would be ill-fated in pots. For best results, choose from the many dwarf varieties with shorter stems and compact foliage, with a base that matures to no more than 1½ feet wide:

> *L. angustifolia* 'Blue Cushion' (a.k.a. 'Schola')
> *L. angustifolia* 'Ellagance' (many colors available)
> *L. angustifolia* 'Lavenite Petite'
> *L. angustifolia* 'Little Lottie' (a.k.a. 'Clarmo')
> *L. angustifolia* 'Nana Alba' (a.k.a. 'Dwarf White')
> *L. angustifolia* 'Thumbelina Leigh'
> *L. angustifolia* 'Wee One'
> *L. stoechas* 'Bandera' (Pink or Purple)
> *L. stoechas* 'Lutsko's Dwarf'
> *L. stoechas* 'Pretty Polly'

COMPANION GARDENING WITH LAVENDER

The fragrance of lavender enhances any sunny garden patch, but lavender's scent can also benefit other garden plants.

ROSES. Place lavender next to roses to attract ladybugs that in turn eat aphids from the roses.

TOMATOES. Set pots of lavender by your tomato plants (or vice versa) to help repel whiteflies.

APPLE AND PEAR TREES. Encircle young trees with lavender to help deter codling moths.

Healing Gardens

Lavender is both an aromatic herb and a flowering shrub, mingling gracefully in herb gardens, cottage gardens, rock gardens, formal gardens, and spice jars. A healing garden with lavender can take up a few square feet—perfect for a sunlit balcony or rooftop oasis—or it can fill an entire yard.

Group together plants that share the same needs for water, sunlight, and temperature. Plant any moisture-lovers downslope of lavender, or consider growing annuals and thirsty plants in pots that you can shelter and water as needed. Here are some companion-garden possibilities.

Herbal Tea Garden

Whether brewed from fresh or dried botanicals, tisanes hold healing properties. Any from this list of aromatics would blend nicely with *L. angustifolia* in herbal teas:

APPLE MINT. Aids digestion. Climate zones 5 to 9. Likes moist soil.

BEE BALM. Relaxing; soothing for fever and nausea. Climate zones 4 to 9.

GINGER. Helps digestion and nausea. Climate zones 7 to 9, evergreen in zones 8 to 9. Water regularly.

LEMON BALM. Relaxing. Climate zones 4 to 9. Likes moist soil.

LEMON THYME. Soothing for cough and sore throat. Climate zones 5 to 9.

PEPPERMINT. Aids digestion. Climate zones 3 to 11. Likes moist soil.

ROMAN CHAMOMILE. Relaxing; soothing for colds. Climate zones 4 to 9. Needs shade in high heat.

ROSEMARY. Supports brain health. Hardiness depends on variety.

TURMERIC. Anti-inflammatory. Climate zones 8 to 11. Likes moist soil.

Edible Flower Garden

For a colorful dose of antioxidants, sprinkle a few petals of edible, organic flowers onto salads and soups, or use them to decorate beverages, desserts, and dinner plates.[2] Be sure to eat only the petals unless you are certain the rest of the blossom is safe to eat, because nonpetal parts of some edible flowers are toxic. Don't eat flowers treated with pesticides. From the rainbow of garden blooms that can be eaten, here are some favorites to complement lavender in an edible flowerbed:

CALENDULA. Bitter flavor. Climate zones 9 to 11 or grow as annuals.

CARNATIONS OR MINIATURE CARNATIONS (*DIANTHUS*). Miniatures fit nicely into pots and rock gardens. Climate zones 3 to 10, depending on variety.

NASTURTIUMS. Peppery flavor. Some varieties are climbers, and others are bushy. Climate zones 9 to 11 or grow as annuals.

PANSIES. Entire flower is edible. Climate zones 4 to 8 or grow as annuals. Needs damp soil.

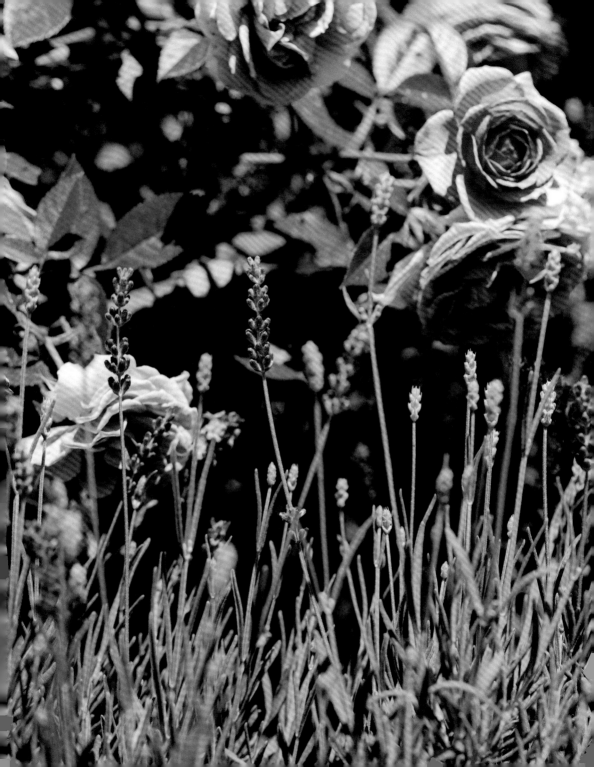

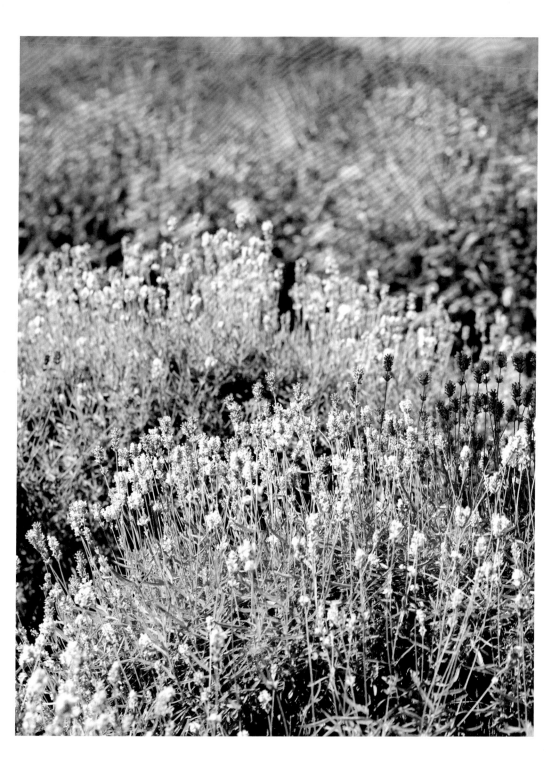

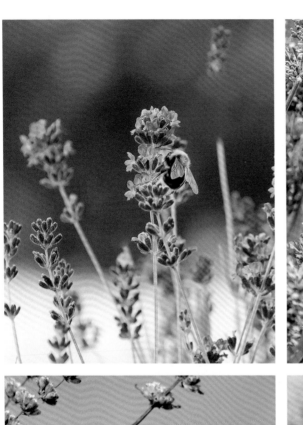
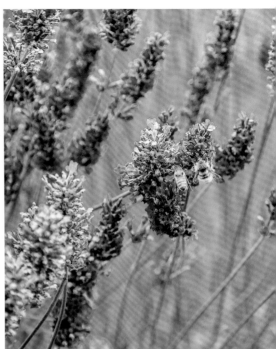
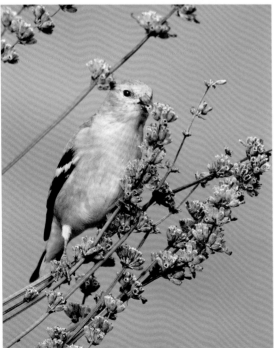
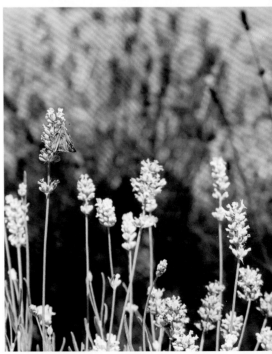

ROSES. Sweet-scented rose petals taste best. Climate and water requirements vary.

SUNFLOWERS. Buds, petals, and seeds are edible. Choose dwarf varieties for small spaces. Climate zones 4 to 9 or grow as annuals.

FLOWERING CULINARY HERBS. Pluck or pinch the flowers from bee balm, chamomile, garlic, oregano, rosemary, sweet marjoram, sage, sweet cicely, or thyme, which all share lavender's drought tolerance. Other flowering herbs, such as basil, borage, chives, dill, mint, and parsley need moist soil and should be planted apart from lavender. Keep rosemary away from all herbs except sage.

Pollinator Garden

Home gardens are vital for pollinators, such as bats, bees, beetles, butterflies, and hummingbirds—especially where homegrown flowers are the only rest stops linking habitat that is fragmented by barren pavement and concrete. A successful pollinator garden depends on several features:

EASY ACCESS FOR POLLINATORS. Choose single-petal blossoms with free access to the flower's nectary. Double-petal and pom-pom blooms (such as pom-pom dahlias) are cultivated to please your eyes, but their dense petals hinder pollinators from gathering food.

Pollinator favorites include stands of open-faced flowers such as hollyhocks, daisies, borage, and *Zinnia*. Other prime choices are clusters of small open flowers such as lavender, sweet alyssum, *Salvia*, *Agastache*, *Origanum*, and *Phlox*.

SUCCESSIVE BLOOMS. Choose plants with overlapping bloom times for an unbroken chain of food for pollinators from early spring through fall. Begin your season with eager plants, such as snowdrops, 'Grace Ward' *Lithodora*, English bluebells, and fruit trees such as purple-leaf plum, apricot, or cherry. Early-blooming *L. angustifolia*s such as 'Folgate', 'Croxton's Wild', and 'Lavenite Petite' will follow in their footsteps. Some late-season blooms that peak during the gap between summer and fall are lavandin, *Hebe*, and the hummingbird-pleaser pineapple sage. Enhance your autumn garden with colorful favorites such as *Sedum* 'Autumn Fire', *Aster*, and sunflowers.

POISON-FREE. Buy organic or wild-crafted plants not treated with neonicotinoid pesticides. Gardens that attract honey-bees to pesticide-laced blooms are dangerous for fragile bee populations. One way to avoid poison is to grow lavender and other plants—such as thyme, nasturtiums, marigolds, and *Allium* such as garlic and chives—that appeal to pollinators but confuse or repel destructive insects.

VARIETY. The nutrients of pollen and nectar vary from plant to plant. To satisfy dietary needs, pollinators visit many differ-ent flowers. Be sure to layer in blooms of different shapes to accommodate all sizes of pollinators.

WATER. A birdbath or fountain will give pollinators a much-needed midday drink. Add a piece of floating wood for bees to rest on too!

Pollinators & Sterile Hybrid Lavandin

In a 2013 bee-counting study at the University of Sussex, 32 garden plants were observed for their attractiveness to insects. Most surprising is that bees preferred the sterile lavandins over the *L. angustifolia*s—possibly because lavandins channel their energy into producing more nectar, while the *L. angustifolia*s divert theirs into growing seed.[3]

Water-Saving Garden

A mingling of drought-tolerant colors, heights, textures, and aromas will be easy on your senses and on your pocketbook. To maximize water savings in arid regions, lay down 2 to 3 inches of natural mulch in the garden to help hold moisture in the soil. Planting next to boulders and stone walls can also provide a cool haven for roots.

Place lavenders behind such rockery companions as creeping thyme, hens and chicks, Cheddar pink (*Dianthus*), and any kind of sedum. Mix your lavenders with Mediterranean herbs, wispy tufted hair grass, swaying poppies, and bright-yellow lavender cotton (*Santolina*). Add striking pops of color with purple coneflowers and black-eyed Susans.

Patio Garden to Repel Flies & Mosquitoes

Some plants carry a scent to deter pesky and biting insects. During warm months, decorate a sunny patio or front-door stoop with large pots of lavender (any variety), rosemary, citronella grass, or lemongrass. Mix them with smaller groupings of aromatic herbs, such as mint, basil, lemon thyme, and sage. Top off your bug barrier with colorful hanging baskets of 'Blue Mink' flossflower, magenta petunias, or trailing rosemary. Note that these plants do attract pollinators, which may include bees and wasps.

Harvest

The perfect time to harvest is when buds are plump and bees are browsing. Depending on the variety of lavender you grow and the end use of your harvest, the timing and steps for cutting may vary, but a few guidelines abide for all lavender: Use sharp, clean tools to enable the plant to heal quickly. Begin harvesting after all morning dew has dried, but not if any rain has fallen in the past 24 hours (dampness will invite fungi to rot your bundles). After harvesting, move bundles out of the sun to preserve flower color and fragrant oil.

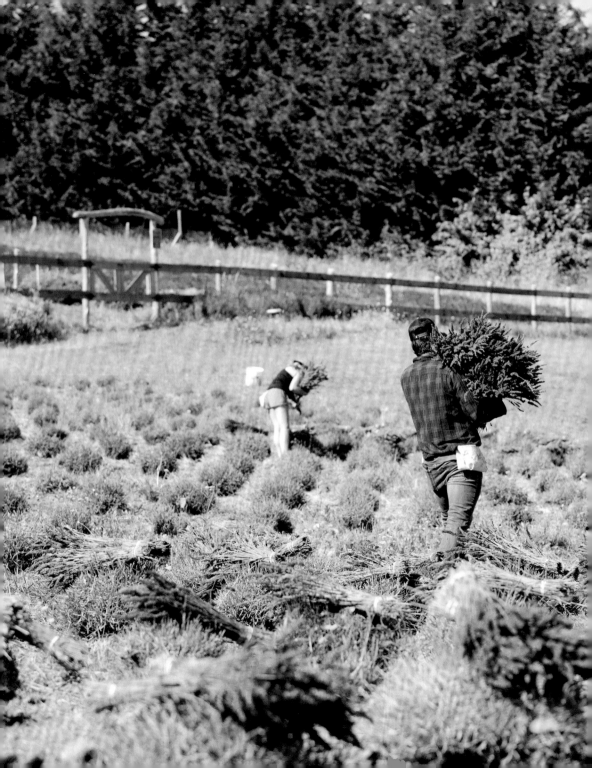

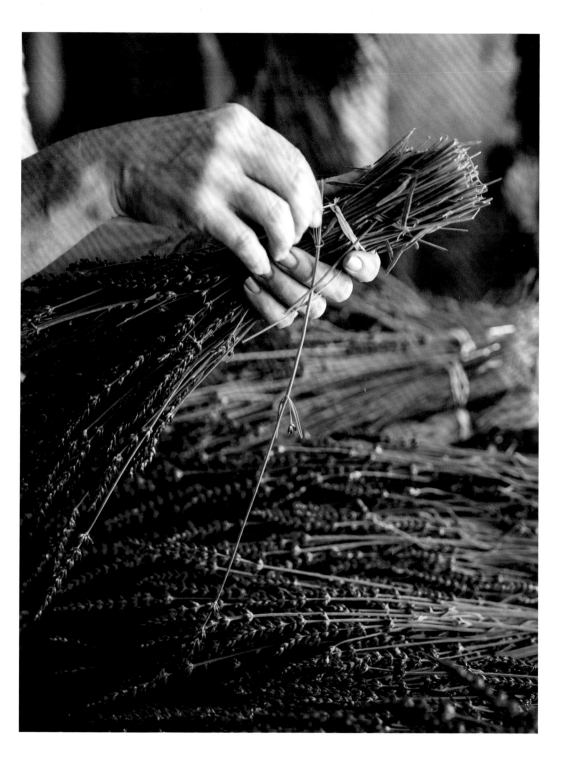

WHEN TO HARVEST

FOR DRIED BUNDLES. Harvest early in the season when the first blossoms open on the plant. This is when the buds cling stubbornly to their stems.

FOR DRIED LOOSE BUDS. If you want clean-looking buds for cooking or because they will be visible in your project, harvest early in the season before the tiny petaled blossoms open and quickly turn brown. If you don't mind a mix of buds and brown withered bits, you can harvest when more of the blossoms have opened. That's when stems easily shed their buds and their wilted blossoms.

FOR FRESH BOUQUETS. Ideally, cut when about half the blooms open. Some buds will continue to blossom after stems are cut.

FOR ESSENTIAL OIL. Wait until most of the blossoms have opened (some will have begun to wither). When harvesting lavender for the purpose of distilling, cut stems only a couple of inches from the flower heads. A little bit of stem is needed to keep flowers from compacting in the still, but too much stem will increase the camphor and decrease the quality of your oil. Later you can go back and prune your plant, and use those bare stalks for fire starters, grilling, or mulch. An interesting study of lavandin revealed that oil production was stimulated by bees removing nectar. In fact, harvesting lavandin after nectar-gathering may increase oil quantity up to 20 percent. The same was not true for L. angustifolia.[1] One study of L. angustifolia showed that its oil quality peaks when temperatures are in the high 70s and no rain has fallen for 10 days before the harvest.[2]

FOR POLLINATORS AND BIRDS. Don't harvest the flowers. Prune at the end of summer, after bees have filled their winter caches and goldfinches have stuffed themselves with seeds. Lavender will be quite dry then, their beds freckled with fallen flowers. Long after you prune the plant, you may see foragers, such as juncos, goldfinch, and towhees, scratching and pecking lavender seed from the ground.

Lavandula angustifolia

If *L. angustifolia* is harvested right after blooming, you may get a second flush of blooms in late summer along with new growth. For this reason, *L. angustifolia* is usually harvested after the spring bloom and later pruned into a mound at the end of the season, around the time of first frost. Several varieties of *L. angustifolia* were cultivated to reliably rebloom, including 'Buena Vista', 'Royal Velvet', 'Sharon Roberts', 'Irene Doyle', 'Tucker's Early Purple', and 'Sachet'. One mature plant should yield about a half dozen handful-sized bundles.

Lavandin

Bursting with nearly a thousand flower heads on each mature plant, lavandin puts on one glorious show a few weeks later in the summer. Prune them into tidy mounds at the same time you harvest their flowers. Given the long stretch of their graceful stems, you'll be cropping off about half the height of the plant all at once. You can expect to harvest about 10 bundles from a mature lavandin.

Lavandula stoechas & Lavandula dentata

Cut flower stalks for use in arrangements and crafts anytime you like. Each stalk you remove stimulates the plant to sprout new flower stems as long as climate permits. Throughout the season, continue to snip out faded blooms. The stem will not rebloom, so when it is finished flowering, go ahead and cut stalks as you would when pruning.

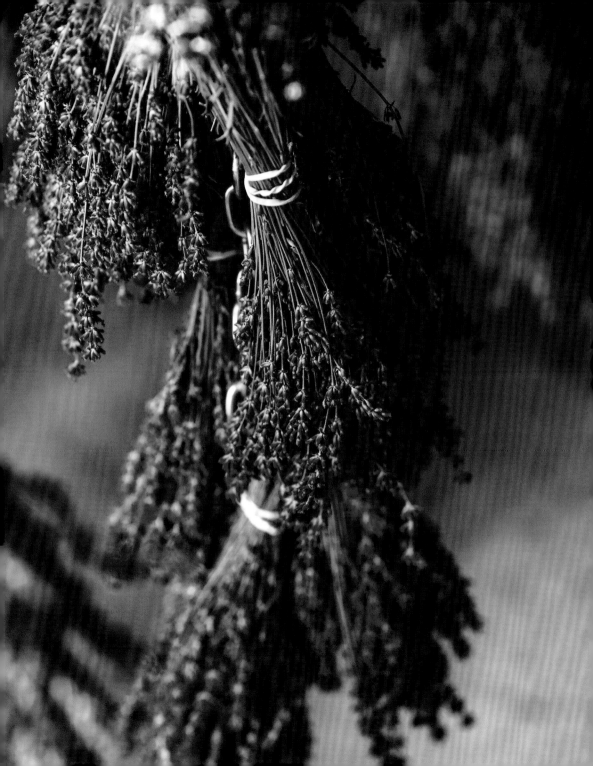

Dried Lavender Bundles & Buds

A perfect drying space is dark, warm, airy, and dry. These conditions are needed because light fades bud color, cool air prolongs drying, and stagnant or humid air allows mold to grow. Don't dry herbs in a garage if they will be exposed to engine or chemical fumes, and avoid oven-drying as excessive heat releases essential oil from flower buds. A fan can help air circulation in places like a dark closet or basement. If you don't have a dim space, loosely tie paper bags around your bundles before drying. Cut a few slits in the bags for airflow, and hang the bags in a dry, ventilated area. Paper bags serve double duty as fallen-bud collectors too.

DRYING THE BUNDLES

Freshly harvested lavender (100 to 200 stalks per bundle)
⅛-inch-by-3-inch rubber bands (1 per bundle)
Ball of twine or hooks
Paper clips (1 per bundle)

• As you harvest, keep rubber bands around your wrist to easily bundle each handful of cut lavender. A couple of inches from the cut ends, girdle the stems a few times with the rubber band, making the band snug but not tight enough to crease the stems. The center of a bundle dries last, so in humid or cool climates, limit the size of each bundle to about 100 stems to help prevent mold. In dry climates with excellent air circulation, bundles of 150 to 200 stems should dry well.

• Hang a taut line of twine in your drying area, long enough to hang bundles side by side, with space for air to flow around each bundle. Make sure the line is strong enough to support the weight of the bundles. If you prefer, hang bundles on a chain, or on individual hooks along a wooden beam, pole, rungs of a wooden ladder, or drying rack.

• Bend the paper clips open to make double-ended hooks.

$\longrightarrow$

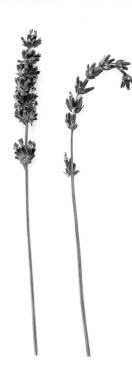

• Attach one end of a paper clip to the rubber band. Use the other end to hang lavender bundles upside down on your twine or hooks.

• It's normal for lavender to shed some buds while drying, so lay a clean sheet under the bundles to collect fallen flowers.

• Bundles should be fully dry within 1 to 6 weeks, depending on drying conditions. Fully dried stems break when bent. If you can fold a stem, it is not yet dry.

• As bundles dry, you may need to tighten rubber bands around shrinking stems. For later use, store dried bundles loosely in a closed cardboard box or paper bag. Keep them in a cool, dark area.

Flower on left: dried hanging upside down
Flower on right: dried standing upright in a vase

FAVORITE VARIETIES FOR DRYING

For best crafting and cooking results, dry the kind of lavender that fits your end use.

FOR STRONG, LASTING FRAGRANCE. In projects where buds are hidden from view, such as the Lavender Bags for Dryers & Drawers (page 111), Soothing Eye Pillow (page 117), or Aromatherapy Wrap with Washable Cover (page 121), scent is more important than appearance.

Lavandula angustifolia. The sweetly scented 'Sachet', bred for its exceptional fragrance, is a popular choice.

Lavandin. Consider the highly fragrant 'Grosso', 'Twickel Purple', or 'Provence'.

FOR RICH COLOR. Many lighter shades of lavender flowers fade to gray when dry. Varieties with the deepest blues or purples retain their colors best, and *L. angustifolia* offers the darkest color choices. Color retention is important when you want to display lavender in salads and desserts, floral arrangements, or in projects such as a Twig & Lavender Wreath (page 125).

Lavandula angustifolia. 'Royal Velvet' and 'Hidcote' are favored for their deep colors. 'Folgate' is often dried for its lighter violet beauty.

Lavandin. 'Gros Bleu' wears richer purple flowers and dries darker than most other lavandins.

FOR LONG STEMS. If your goal is bouquets or wands, opt for long-stemmed varieties. Lavandins offer the longest stems and strongest fragrance.

Lavandula angustifolia. 'Buena Vista', 'Royal Velvet', and 'Sharon Roberts' have been bred to produce stems as long as 10 to 16 inches when grown in ideal conditions.

Lavandin. Stem length of most lavandins ranges from 16 to 24 inches. You'll find extra-long stems on varieties such as 'Hidcote Giant', 'Super', 'Seal', 'Dutch Mill', and 'Edelweiss'. The bright-white blooms of 'Edelweiss' will fade but still add a nice contrast to bouquets.

FOR CULINARY USE. See Culinary Lavender (page 132).

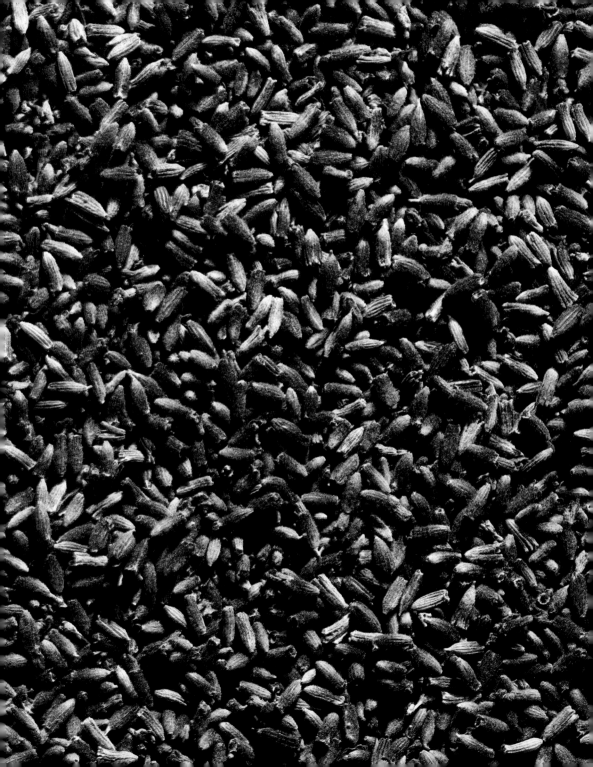

Removing Dried Lavender Buds

Dried lavender bundles
2 large bowls or tubs
1 large ⅛-inch-mesh
    screen or strainer
    (optional)
1 large fine-mesh screen
    or sieve (optional)

• To remove buds from their stalks, hold a bunch of lavender stalks over a large tub or bowl and gently bump the flower heads against the side of the tub. To remove any remaining stubborn buds from the stalks, pinch your thumb and finger over a stalk of lavender and slide your fingers to the end, scraping the flowers from the stem as you go. With fingers or tweezers, pick out any sharp stem pieces from the bowl of buds. When buds will be hidden inside pouches or pillows, this is all you need to do.

• When buds will be visible in your craft or cooking project, you'll want to sift the buds. Set a ⅛-inch-mesh strainer over an empty bowl. Pour lavender buds into the strainer, and gently run your hand back and forth over the flowers on the screen until buds have all dropped through to the bowl. Discard remaining pieces of stem. Repeat and pick out any big pieces of stem that slipped through the holes. Repeat again with a fine-mesh sieve. This time the clean buds will remain in the strainer while the dust and tiny debris pass through.

• Your buds may still contain particles of wilted lavender litter from the dried flower bracts. They're not harmful, but if you want an especially pretty batch of buds, here's a trick: Lightweight lavender litter is attracted to plastic by static electricity. Pour your buds into a plastic container, close the lid, and give the container a few shakes (if needed, rub the inside of the lid with your fingers to increase static electricity). When you remove the lid, lightweight particles will cling to the lid. Repeat if needed.

• Keep dried buds in a cool, dark area. For culinary use, loose buds keep best in airtight glass jars. For craft use, buds can be stored in resealable bags.

Essence

While no herb can guarantee cure or relief, and researchers don't fully understand the complexities of essential oil, nearly every study points in the same direction—that certain components of lavender oil genuinely and significantly help some people. You might benefit from using lavender oil in one of these ways:

Bath. To enhance a warm bath and help relax tensions, sore muscles, and aching joints.

Compress. To boost the benefits of a hot or cold compress. A hot compress can help with localized muscle pain, tension headaches, menstrual cramps, earaches, or toothaches. A cold compress can help soothe headaches, inflamed joints, muscles, and insect bites.

Diffuser. To help soothe coughing and colds, anxiety, or sleep troubles.

Massage. To increase the relaxing or therapeutic effects of a localized or full-body massage.

Steam. To gently support facial skin or to help relieve congestion and coughing.

Topical. To help soothe insect bites or stings, minor cuts or burns, and tension-related headaches.

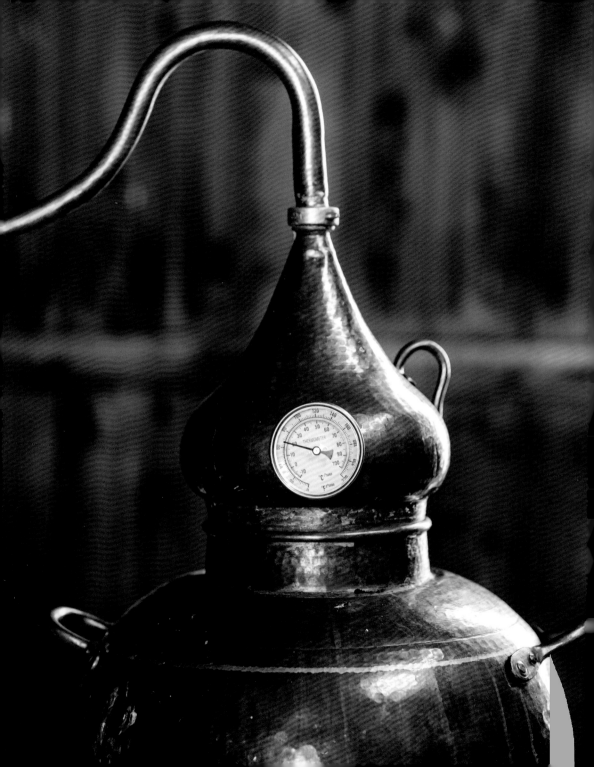

WHY DO FLOWERS MAKE OIL & WHY IS IT ESSENTIAL?

The word *essential* in modern English means that something is absolutely necessary. *Essential* in the context of an essential amino or fatty acid means that your body needs it, can't produce it, and must get it from food. But in the Middle Ages *essential* also meant something different.

Paracelsus, who was a brilliant but highly unconventional sixteenth-century doctor, wrote, "The quinta essentia is that which is extracted from a substance—from all plants and from everything which has life—then freed of all impurities and all perishable parts, refined into highest purity and separated from all elements."[1] He was describing the *essence* of living things. Thanks to Paracelsus, *essential* oil came to mean the essence extracted from a plant.

The essence of a plant is a complex and unique blend of living chemistry. It often holds a scent that appeals to pollinators and repels predators. Many studies have shown that some essential oils also hold natural components that are able to destroy specific bacteria or fungi. Because plants cannot run away from threats, it makes sense that they'd possess some means to defend against invading pathogens. And those pathogens are often the same ones that threaten you.

Around the globe, lavender essential oil is the subject of many studies, each one searching for reliable ways to harness the powerful defenses hidden within lavender oil. The oil is being tested—with hope and excitement—for its potential as a nonaddictive painkiller and antianxiety medication, and for its ability to compound with other natural elements in the fight against cancerous tumors and drug-resistant germs.[2] Much remains to be explored, but from existing chemical, physiological, and psychological research, some promising results have emerged.

CHOOSING THE RIGHT LAVENDER OIL

For relaxation, one species of lavender is most recommended by aromatherapists. *Lavandula angustifolia* has a sweet, floral scent with scarcely any of the sharp, invigorating scent of camphor found in other species.[3] Lavandin oil is more aromatic and can be beneficial when used for purposes that fit the chemical profile of the oil, such as germ-fighting, muscle stiffness, and chest congestion. Lower-camphor varieties of lavandin are less penetrating and hold stronger soothing properties.

When following an aromatherapy recipe, don't substitute any other essential oil for lavender oil, and don't substitute one lavender species for another. Some lavenders are higher in camphor and/or eucalyptol. Camphor has antibacterial properties, is a stimulant, and is penetrating. When highly diluted, it's useful in treating congestion and coughs. But camphor levels above 11 percent are linked to seizures and poisoning.[4] Eucalyptol has potent antibacterial and anti-inflammatory properties but is also a stimulant with higher risk of skin irritation and seizures.[5]

EVERY BATCH OF ESSENTIAL OIL IS UNIQUE

The oil within each harvest of lavender is a blend of hundreds of active chemical compounds. Unlike prescription drugs that are synthesized and regulated so that each dose is precisely identical, essential oils maintain the natural biodiversity of a plant that adapts and responds to its environment in its mission to survive and reproduce. As with all flora, the essences of lavender change from year to year and place to place.

Methods of growing, harvesting, handling, and extracting also create significant differences in the oils. For example, testing shows that the highest-quality lavender oils are produced using carbon dioxide (CO_2) extraction and steam distillation.[6]

Oils from *L. angustifolia* plants in different parts of the world reveal startling inconsistencies. In a couple of tests from Iran and Brazil, two key chemical compounds, linalool and linalyl acetate, were completely absent from the batches tested. Studies show that these key components appear to be the elements responsible for soothing anxiety[7] and reducing inflammation.[8] In some tests from China, Greece, and Syria, linalool was present but linalyl acetate was not found.[9] The *L. angustifolia* oil from Iran also held more than 10 times the standard amount of camphor.[10]

Chemical inconsistencies like these can greatly alter an oil's potential benefits. To some degree, every batch of essential oil will have a unique chemical balance, and that unpredictability has hindered global researchers from producing consistent clinical results.

International standards specify the basic chemical makeup that each type of lavender oil should contain. When buying lavender oil, you can ask to see the gas chromatography–mass spectrometry (GC-MS) report for that batch of oil. The report is long and mystifying, but just focus on a few key ingredients to see if the oil meets these key standards:

	L. ANGUSTIFOLIA	LAVANDIN
Linalyl acetate	at least 20%	at least 20%
Linalool	at least 20%	at least 20%
Eucalyptol (1,8-cineole)	up to 3%	up to 12%
Camphor	up to 1%	up to 12%

Essential Oil versus Infused Oil

Confusingly, lavender essential oil and lavender-infused oil are both called *lavender oil*. In this book, any reference to *lavender oil* infers *essential*. Lavender-infused oil will not be abbreviated.

Lavender-infused oil is a simple fragrant steeping of lavender in a neutral oil, which produces a scented oil without the potency or health benefits of essential oil. Making lavender-infused oil is easy! For a recipe, see Lavender-Infused Oils & Vinegars on page 144. Lavender-infused oil is useful in all kinds of recipes and do-it-yourself beauty products.

Making essential oil, however, is lengthy and exacting, especially for therapeutic use. You could distill your own essential oil with a glass microwave kit, a jury-rigged tea kettle, a stainless-steel pressure cooker, or a copper still, but you might be quite disappointed by the quantity and quality of your oil. It's a fun experiment, and some may enjoy the deep dive into the details of the process (it's comparable to distilling alcohol), but for aromatherapy the safest option is to purchase essential oil from a trusted source.

FAVORITE LAVENDER VARIETIES FOR ESSENTIAL OIL

The search for the perfect lavender oil has led to hundreds of cultivated varieties of lavender, all in pursuit of exceptional oil quantity and fragrance quality. If you choose to distill your own lavender oil, here are some favorite varieties to grow or harvest:

Lavandula angustifolia essential oil is most commonly used for cooking, perfume, and aromatherapy. 'Folgate', 'Maillette', 'Buena Vista', and 'Hidcote' are a few of the more popular varieties grown for pleasing fragrance profiles and a higher number of buds per stem.

Lavandin produces more buds and more oil per plant. It is most used in crafts, air fresheners, candles, soap, cleaning products, and insect repellents. Worldwide, 70 percent of all lavender oil comes from the oil-rich lavandin *L.* x *intermedia* 'Grosso'. Other popular lavandin oil producers are 'Super', 'Hidcote Giant', 'Phenomenal', 'Impress Purple', and 'Provence'.

HOW TO STORE LAVENDER OIL

Essential oils are volatile. *Volatile* in this sense doesn't imply *dangerous*. It means that the chemical components of the oil evaporate easily at room temperature. When carefully stored, the bioactive properties of your lavender oil should last 1 to 2 years. To ensure the life span of essential oil, protect it from these degrading elements:

LIGHT. Store oil in a dark-colored glass bottle away from sunlight. Light of any kind reacts with an oil's compounds. Amber glass offers the most protection, followed by cobalt glass.

PLASTICS AND METALS. Use glass containers, which don't alter the properties of essential oil.

HEAT. Oxidation is slowest when lavender oil is refrigerated.[11] The warmer the ambient temperature, the more quickly essential oil will degrade.

MOISTURE. Keep bottles tightly closed to prevent humidity from interacting with oils.

OXYGEN. Exposure to air can weaken antibacterial activity and cause contact allergens to develop.[12] Use small bottles to reduce headspace and minimize oxidation.[13]

Be sure to buy fresh lavender oil. You can inquire about the manufacture or best-by date to avoid oils that have been sitting on shop shelves for too long.

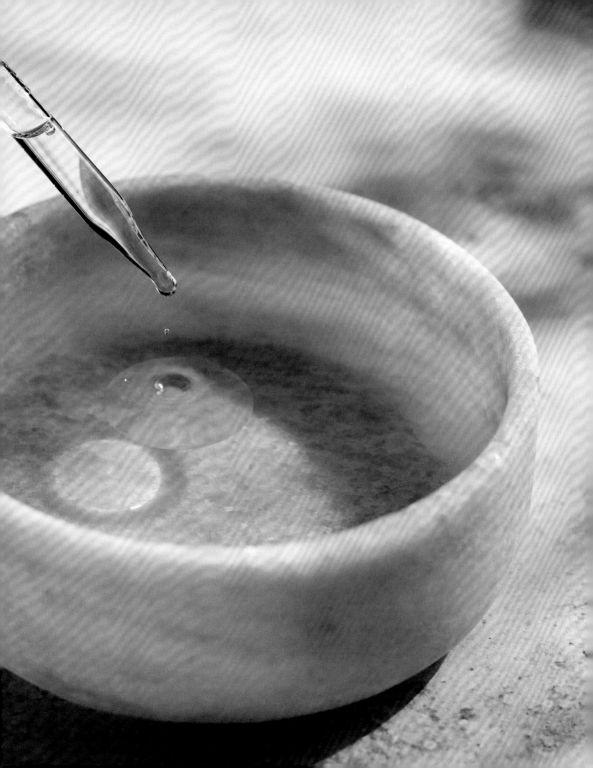

ESSENTIAL OIL DILUTION

Essential oils are so concentrated that it takes all the flowers from an entire *L. angustifolia* plant to produce a single teaspoon of essential oil! Applying most oils undiluted (called "neat") can cause severe reactions, but diluting essential oil lets you to cover a much larger area of your body without using a toxic or wasteful amount of oil. The renowned father of aromatherapy, René-Maurice Gattefossé, came to a notable conclusion after 30 years of working with essential oils: "It is totally futile to use the pure essences. The same dynamic effects on cells are obtained at a high dilution."[14]

Lavandula angustifolia is one of the few oils that may be applied neat, but only to nonsensitized adult skin in tiny, occasional doses. Using lavender oil in high quantity or for an extended time greatly increases the risk of developing a sensitivity to chemical components in the oil.

You can safely dilute essential oils with specific carriers (see Dilution Guidelines on page 58 and Popular Essential Oil Carriers on page 60). The carrier's job is to disperse and deliver components of the essential oil safely to your skin, where they can be absorbed into your bloodstream. Most carriers are mild oils with little or no scent. Another effective carrier is Natrasorb Bath, which is a uniquely modified tapioca starch that doesn't leave an oily film in the tub. Essential oils cannot be diluted in water because they are hydrophobic. Like unshaken vinaigrette, the oils float atop the bathwater—where the sensitive parts of your body that first contact the water can get the full and potentially dangerous impact of undiluted essential oil.

Allergic reactions to carriers are possible, so patch-testing is recommended. If you have a nut allergy, do not use any nut or kernel oils.

The Size of a Drop Is Unique

When exact ratios are needed for blending oils, measuring is done by weight. But since personal users rarely own a scale that is accurate to a fraction of a gram, measuring for small recipes is typically done by counting drops. For best results, consistently use one brand of dropper for all oils in a recipe.

DILUTION GUIDELINES

	1%	2%	3%	5%	10+%
	Adult facial skin; adults with mature or sensitive skin, impaired immune systems, or serious health problems	Most adults with normal skin; for massage or skin care	Most adults with normal skin; for short-term support with minor pain or congestion	Most adults with normal skin; only for short-term use on acute muscle pain or cramping	With a doctor's supervision; only for short-term use with acute issues
1 teaspoon 5 milliliters ⅙ ounce	1 ◆	2 ◆	3 ◆	5 ◆	
2 teaspoons 10 milliliters ⅓ ounce	2 ◆	4 ◆	6 ◆	10 ◆	Only as directed by your doctor
1 tablespoon 15 milliliters ½ ounce	3 ◆	6 ◆	9 ◆	15 ◆	
¼ cup 60 milliliters 2 ounces	12 ◆	24 ◆	36 ◆	60 ◆	

For oil-based carriers, consider these tips:

- On the label, look for the words *organic*, *unprocessed*, *unrefined*, *extra virgin*, *cold pressed*, or for coconut oil, *fractionated*. Avoid oils that have been processed with chemicals and/or nutrient-destroying heat. Also avoid oils with preservatives and oils labeled *hydrogenated* or *vegetable oil*.
- Organic, unrefined oils cost more and have a shorter shelf life. Buy in small bottles that you can keep refrigerated.

- Saturated-fat carriers (like shea butter, cocoa butter, and unrefined coconut oil) sit atop the skin instead of absorbing into the skin. They block moisture loss, but they also block skin pores. Limit to sparing, occasional use.

SYNERGY OF BLENDED OILS

Centuries of traditional healers have blended essential oils to create synergy, which is the effect produced when chemical elements interact. Blending is still popular today, and much essential oil synergy can be explained by science.[15] Not all synergy is good, though. Positive synergy is when the whole is greater than the sum of its parts. But negative synergy is equally possible. When blended oils antagonize each other, benefits are dampened or destroyed.

Before getting creative with blends on your own, seek out a trained aromatherapist who understands the potential benefits, vulnerabilities, and dangers of each essential oil and the synergies created by blending. Draw from their wealth of experience and allow them to guide you toward blends of oils that match your individual needs.

Here are a few basic guidelines aromatherapists use to create harmonious synergy and avoid a malodorous stew:

- Start with 1 drop. Adding drops is easy; removing them is impossible.
- Mix and allow the blend to settle for at least 5 minutes. The overall fragrance will change as top notes fade and base notes develop.
- Simple synergy is effective. Choose 3 to 5 oils but no more than 7 oils.
- For balance, use fewer drops of the oils that have powerful, lingering scents. Use more drops of milder oils.

Popular Essential Oil Carriers

	SCENT	ABSORPTION	SKIN TYPE	USES	REFRIGERATED SHELF LIFE
Almond oil, sweet	Mild	Average, leaves slight oily residue	Sensitive, itchy, oily, combination. Caution: tree nut allergen	Massage & bath oil, lotion, hair care, wood polish	3–12 months
Apricot kernel oil	Mild	Fast, moisturizes with no residue	Sensitive, dry, mature, acne. Caution: tree nut allergen	All-purpose	3–12 months
Avocado oil	Mild	Slow, leaves oily residue	Dry, mature, eczema, psoriasis, sun-damaged Caution: latex allergen	Dry patches only, or mix with a lighter carrier oil	1–3 years
Coconut oil, fractionated (liquid)	Unscented	Average, leaves satiny residue	Sensitive, dry	All-purpose short-term, may clog pores	4–5 years
Coconut oil, unrefined (solid)	Strong	Very slow, leaves thick oily residue	Very dry, sunburned, eczema, psoriasis	Can clog pores, short-term use for extra-dry patches	2–5 years
Flaxseed oil	Strong	Slow, leaves oily residue	Sensitive, dry, mature, inflamed, eczema, psoriasis	Joint & foot massages, lotion, hair care	3–12 months
Grapeseed oil	Mild	Fast, moisturizes with no residue	All, including oily, combination, mature, acne	All-purpose	3–12 months

	SCENT	ABSORPTION	SKIN TYPE	USES	REFRIGERATED SHELF LIFE
Jojoba oil	Mild	Average, leaves satiny residue	All, including rosacea, eczema, psoriasis, acne	All-purpose	3–5 years
Olive oil, extra virgin	Strong	Slow, leaves oily residue	Dry, mature, inflamed, rosacea, eczema, psoriasis	All-purpose when mixed with milder carrier oil	2–3 years
Sunflower oil, low oleic acid	Mild	Average, leaves light oily residue	All, including eczema, psoriasis. Caution: ragweed allergen	All-purpose	2 years
Cocoa butter	Medium	Slow, leaves oily residue	Sun-damaged, dry, sunburned. Not for oily skin.	Lip balm, sun care, body butter, soap; brittle when cool	1–2 years
Mango butter	Mild	Fast, moisturizes with little residue	All, including rough, dry, mature	Lotion, lip balm, body butter, hair care, soap	3–12 months
Lotion/cream, natural	Unscented	Very fast, no oily residue	All skin types	All-purpose, good for deep tissue massage	1–2 years
Natrasorb Bath	Unscented	N/A (modified tapioca starch), no residue	All skin types	Bath	2 years (no refrigeration needed)

Body

From east to west, from ancient eras to modern days, for young and old, and for men and women, droplets of lavender oil have undoubtedly lessened pain, soothed headaches, and helped heal wounds. Although results can vary among users, lavender's potential benefits cannot be denied.

Consider that your body itself is unique, and then factor in your physical activity, stress level, ailments, prescriptions, diet, biases, and moods. All these contribute to how you respond to treatment, whether it be pharmaceutical or natural. If one natural blend or method doesn't help, don't give up. Another just might work.

MUSCLE RELAXATION

Current research suggests that lavender essential oil high in linalool and linalyl acetate, such as *L. angustifolia*, has the potential to induce relaxation, decrease inflammation, and lessen pain.[1] If you hold stress in your neck and shoulders and suffer from tension headaches, or if you hold anxiety in the belly and then cope with digestion issues, this is hopeful news. Lavender oil absorbed into the skin may help those causal muscles to relax.[2]

PAIN MANAGEMENT

Although recent studies pose new questions, a body of evidence is growing in support of lavender aromatherapy for pain. In some studies, diluted lavender oil applied directly to a painful area has lessened pain from joints and wounds.[3] Some clinical trials in the Middle East concluded that inhaled lavender oil may decrease perception of post-surgery pain[4] as well as the severity of labor pains.[5] In another study, head-aches responded either partially or completely to inhalation of the oil.[6] In other recent tests, therapeutic doses of lavender essential oil helped mice with neuropathic and inflammatory pain without addictive or behavioral side effects.[7]

ANTIOXIDANT BOOST

Lavender oil contains antioxidants known to help protect the body from oxidative stress, which is a factor in such major diseases as diabetes, heart disease, and cancer. For example, one way that stress creates oxidative wear and tear on the body is by elevating cortisol—the body's fight-or-flight hormone. Cortisol levels can be measured in the saliva, and an interesting study in Japan showed that inhaling lavender oil for 5 minutes immediately decreased salivary cortisol levels.[8]

TOPICAL WOUND TREATMENT

Lavender oil has been shown to accelerate the regeneration of tissue, especially when applied immediately to a minor topical wound. It may calm inflammation and hasten healing of cuts, scratches, ulcers, blisters, stings, and surface burns. Studies also report a mildly anesthetic effect that lessens the pain of these topical wounds.[9]

Lavender's Colorful History

The esteemed herb would be nothing less than magical if all of history's curative claims were true. In *The Complete Herbal* published in 1653, Dr. Nicholas Culpeper offered this eyebrow-raising advice:

> *Lavender is of a special good use for all the griefs and pains of the head and brain that proceed of a cold cause, as the apoplexy, falling-sickness, the dropsy, or sluggish malady, cramps, convulsions, palsies, and often faintings. It strengthens the stomach, and frees the liver and spleen from obstructions, provokes women's courses, and expels the dead child and after-birth.*[10]

Before you consider running with Dr. Culpeper's advice, you may want to know that he died at the age of 37, and only 1 of his 7 children lived to reach adulthood.

As science advanced, traditional medicine gave way to modern pharmacology, which branded many natural botanical treatments as superstition. But our understanding of lavender has come a long way. Within every drop of lavender oil, bioactive properties interact, and by assaying those active ingredients, science has been solidly piecing together verifiable healing benefits.

Muscle-Soothing Massage Oil

Enhance the relief of a massage with soothing essential oils. Each essential oil within this blend contains a component with some promising clinical effectiveness against either pain, inflammation, or both.

½ cup organic sweet almond oil
½ cup jojoba oil
30 drops black spruce essential oil
21 drops *L. angustifolia* lavender essential oil
21 drops sweet orange essential oil
9 drops frankincense essential oil
6 drops sandalwood essential oil
1 (8-ounce) amber or cobalt glass bottle

MAKES 8 OUNCES

◆ In a glass pitcher or measuring cup with a spout, mix the almond and jojoba oils.

◆ With a spoon, gently stir the essential oils into the carrier-oil mixture.

◆ Pour the massage oil blend into the bottle.

◆ Store in a cool, dark place. Keep out of reach of children.

TO USE: Place a few drops of massage oil into your hand, and rub your palms together to warm the oil. Apply to skin with the massage technique of your choice.

Note: When a recipe in this book calls for many drops of an essential oil, don't worry about an extra drop or two. The fragrance will change slightly, but you don't need to start over for the sake of safety.

Germ-Slaying Salve

Lavender, tea tree, and lemon all possess antimicrobial properties, each effective against different groups of organisms. Here they join forces to help heal minor cuts and scratches.

2½ teaspoons ethically harvested, filtered organic beeswax pellets

1 tablespoon extra-virgin olive oil

1 tablespoon virgin (unrefined) coconut oil

3 drops lavandin essential oil

3 drops tea tree essential oil

3 drops lemon essential oil

1 (1-ounce) flat metal tin or glass container

MAKES 1 OUNCE

✦ Before you begin, review the Wax-Melting Safety Tips below. In the top of a double boiler over low heat, melt the beeswax, olive oil, and coconut oil together. (Alternatively, melt the ingredients in a clean metal can or pitcher set into a pan of simmering water.) Remove from heat.

✦ Add the essential oils and stir all the ingredients together.

✦ Slowly pour the mixture into the container and allow to harden, 4 to 8 hours.

✦ Store in a cool, dark place. Keep out of reach of children.

TO USE: Apply as needed.

Wax-Melting Safety Tips

Don't use high heat or a microwave.

Use a double-boiler method with water in the bottom pan.

Don't leave melting wax unattended on the stove top.

Be careful not to splash wax onto the stove top or yourself.

In case of fire, keep a bag of baking soda handy. (Water accelerates a wax fire!)

Don't wash wax down the drain.

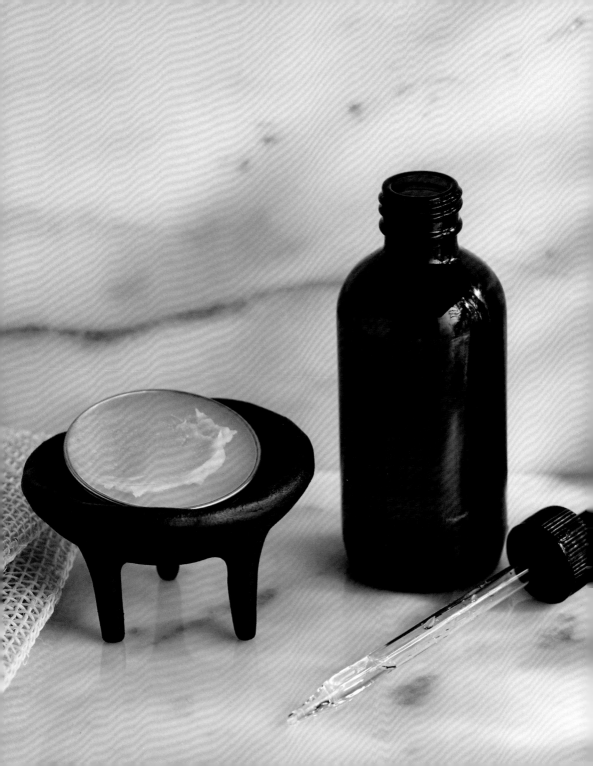

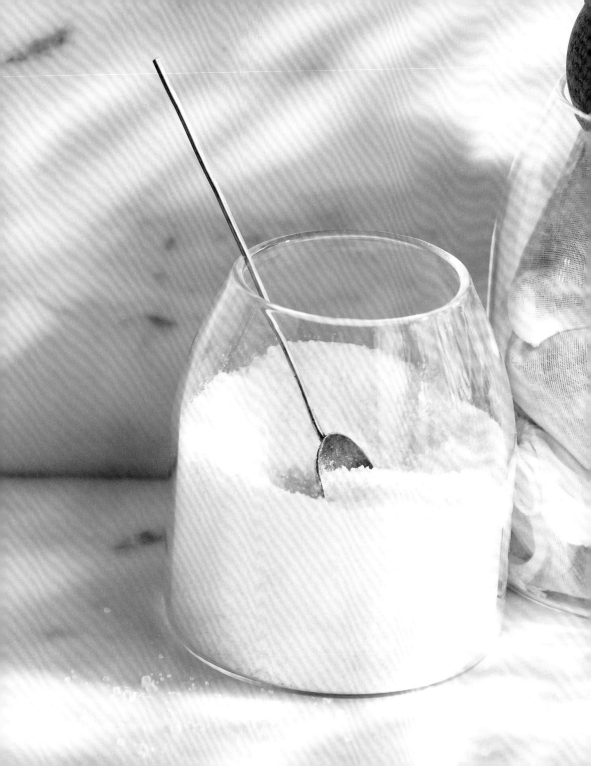

Congestion-Loosening Steam

Combined with rising heat and moisture from steaming water, this blend can help open stuffy airways. Be sure to keep some tissues handy during the process! You can also use a few drops of the blend in an aromatherapy inhaler or diffuser, but not directly on skin.

1 (5-milliliter) amber or cobalt glass bottle

15 drops *Eucalyptus radiata* essential oil

10 drops Siberian fir essential oil

5 drops *L. angustifolia* lavender essential oil

3 drops tea tree essential oil

MAKES ENOUGH FOR 15 TO 30 USES

+ In the bottle, combine essential oils and cap tightly.

+ Store in a cool, dark place. Keep out of reach of children.

TO USE: Into a heatproof bowl, pour 1 quart of boiling water. Shake the bottle gently before use. Add 1 to 2 drops of the oil blend to the water. Lean over the bowl and close your eyes to prevent irritation. Cover your head and the bowl with a large towel. Breathe through your nose as much as possible for 5 minutes, taking fresh-air breaks as needed. Be careful to approach steam very slowly, and pull away anytime it feels too hot or if you feel light-headed.

Foot-Revitalizing Soak

Immerse tired, achy feet in a bath of healing mineral salt and sensory oils. For gifting a jar of soaking salts, use ribbon to attach a small wooden spoon, instructions, and a snip of lavender.

2 tablespoons Natrasorb Bath, or 1 tablespoon almond, olive, or jojoba oil

8 drops sweet orange essential oil

8 drops *L. angustifolia* lavender essential oil

5 drops frankincense essential oil

1 cup US Pharmacopeia (USP)–approved Epsom salt

1 (8-ounce) glass jar with airtight lid

MAKES ENOUGH FOR 3 USES

◆ In a small glass bowl, combine the Natrasorb and oils. Use a fork to mix well.

◆ Add Epsom salt, mix again, and transfer to the jar.

◆ Keep the jar tightly closed to protect from moisture. Keep out of reach of children.

TO USE: Fill a foot-soaking tub with warm water. Add ⅓ cup of the mixture and stir gently to dissolve the salt crystals. Soak feet for 15 to 20 minutes. Rinse feet and pat dry.

Sunburn-Cooling Spray

Hydrosol is the floral or herbal water that is naturally created as a by-product when essential oil is extracted from plants during steam distillation. Lavender combines here with peppermint and aloe vera to cool painful, heat-radiating skin after too much sun (or a minor burn).

1 (4-ounce) amber or cobalt bottle with sprayer
¼ cup aloe vera gel
2 tablespoons L. angustifolia hydrosol
2 tablespoons peppermint hydrosol

MAKES 4 OUNCES

◆ In the bottle, combine the aloe vera gel and hydrosols.

◆ Cap tightly, shake to mix, and store in a cool, dark place. For shelf-life guidelines, see How to Store Lavender Oil on page 55.

TO USE: Shake before use. Spray on affected areas as needed.

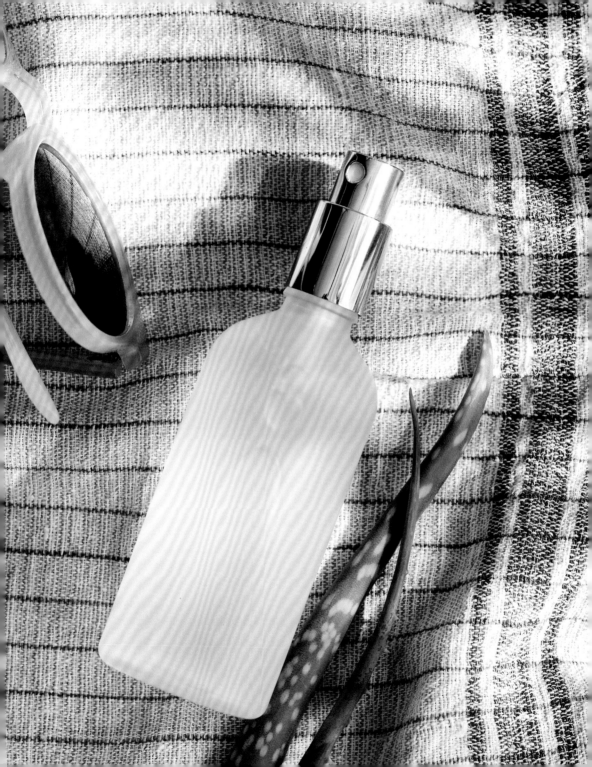

Mind

For centuries people have inhaled lavender oil to help with anxiety, agitation, insomnia, and depression. Today we know that aromatherapy is much more than enjoying a pleasing fragrance. It's a way for chemical molecules to access your bloodstream. And it's the bloodstream that transports lavender's bioactive properties to the central nervous system and throughout the body.[1]

So what happens during aromatherapy if you've lost your sense of smell? Or what if the fragrance you're diffusing reminds you of a depressing funeral? Researchers are finally unraveling these and other intriguing mysteries behind aromatherapy.

THE SENSE OF SMELL

A notable study in Japan divided a group of women into two clusters: those who liked and those who disliked the scent of lavender. Electrical leads were attached to the women's scalps, and the women were asked to inhale lavender essential oil. For the women who liked the scent, EEG readings showed a significant change in their alpha-1 waves, while the other group showed little brain-wave change.[2]

Changes in these brain waves link directly to a person's perception of pain or comfort.[3] The Japanese researchers concluded that an intense emotional response to an unpleasant odor can overpower the alpha-1 brain-wave change. So it is entirely possible that enjoying a scent could boost the positive effects of an essential oil for you, whereas disliking the scent could negate nearly all its benefits.

Dr. Foveau de Courmelles, a colleague of René-Maurice Gattefossé, the father of aromatherapy, once mused about the possibility of therapeutic benefits of smells: "Which are the best? The ones we prefer."[4]

Some aromatherapy research has focused on the direct path from the nose to the olfactory bulb to the brain's amygdala. The amygdala is part of the limbic system that gets input from your sense of smell, along with other senses, and helps your brain process and respond to emotions.

Clinical trials for anxiety have produced inconsistent but promising results.[5] The inconsistency is partly because the effects of aromatherapy may be skewed by scent triggers embedded in your memory. For example, lavender's fragrance may transport your mind to a peaceful garden under a flawless blue sky. Or it might remind you of the warmth of your grandmother's lap. On the other hand, the scent may flood you with impressions of a dank and musty secondhand shop.

But most interesting are two separate studies in Japan and Brazil. The relaxing effects of inhaled lavender oil were tested on groups of mice with and without a sense of smell. Surprisingly, the same calming of anxiety was observed in both groups of mice. These results led the research teams to conclude that no detection of scent was needed at all to produce the calming benefits of lavender oil. They determined that inhaled molecules of linalool and linalyl acetate are absorbed by the inner lining of the respiratory tract, which is a gateway to the bloodstream.[6]

In both groups—with and without the ability to smell—the serotonin changes and the easing of anxiety were remarkably similar to another control group that was injected with the antianxiety medication diazepam. While this is still unconfirmed in humans, it's believed that inhaled components of lavender oil can reach the human central nervous system even for those without a sense of smell.

In other words, if you enjoy smelling lavender, there's a good chance you'll benefit from lavender reaching your bloodstream via aromatherapy. And if you don't like the scent of lavender, you'll likely have better results if you hide a drop or two on the bottoms of your feet, where your perception of the scent won't cancel out the benefits of the oil.

LAVENDER OIL MASSAGE

It is well known that massage can induce relaxation on its own, but many people claim that lavender aromatherapy increases the calming benefit of their massage. The skin is another pathway for lavender's chemical properties to enter the bloodstream, and research has shown that traces of linalool and linalyl acetate may reach the bloodstream within minutes. Sufficient absorption by the skin could contribute to the relaxing and sedative effects of *L. angustifolia*.[7]

How much and how quickly your skin absorbs the components of lavender oil will vary. Chemicals are absorbed more readily by skin that is thin, damaged, warm, clean, moisturized, very young, postmenopausal, or shaven. Absorption is slower into skin that is chilly, dirty, dry, or hairy.

The part of your body where you apply essential oil makes a difference too. One study revealed a few body parts that have higher and lower absorption rates. Ranking from fastest to slowest in absorption are forehead, armpit, scalp, back, abdomen, palms, and soles of feet.[8] Even with the slowest absorption, foot soles remain a popular aromatherapy point, especially for applying oils with a strong scent or that may cause irritation in thinner-skinned areas.

LAVENDER OIL CAPSULES

Capsules of standardized *L. angustifolia* oil have been shown to help with anxiety, depression, and insomnia with no risk of addiction. At the time of this writing, it appears that the studies most strongly supporting this claim were funded by the makers of over-the-counter lavender oil capsules. That presents a question of funding bias. If swallowing lavender capsules interests you, carefully research the subject, talk it over with your physician, and then make an informed decision.[9]

Bright Moments To Go

Whether you're on the go or staying in place, it takes only a moment to apply a few swirls of this energizing blend of oils. For a gentle energy lift at home, make this blend without the carrier oil and use it in a room diffuser instead.

1 (10-milliliter) glass roll-on bottle

7 drops grapefruit essential oil

4 drops lavandin essential oil

3 drops sweet orange essential oil

3 drops *Eucalyptus radiata* essential oil

2 drops peppermint essential oil

2 teaspoons fractionated coconut oil

MAKES ABOUT 20 APPLICATIONS

• In the bottle, combine the essential oils. Swirl gently to blend.

• Add the coconut oil, cap tightly, and shake to mix.

• Store the bottle in a cool, dark place. Keep out of reach of children.

TO USE: In a circular motion, apply to the sides of the neck and the pulse point on each wrist. Inhale deeply. Apply up to 3 times a day. To use the blend in a diffuser, omit the coconut oil. Add 5 to 6 drops to a diffuser for each use.

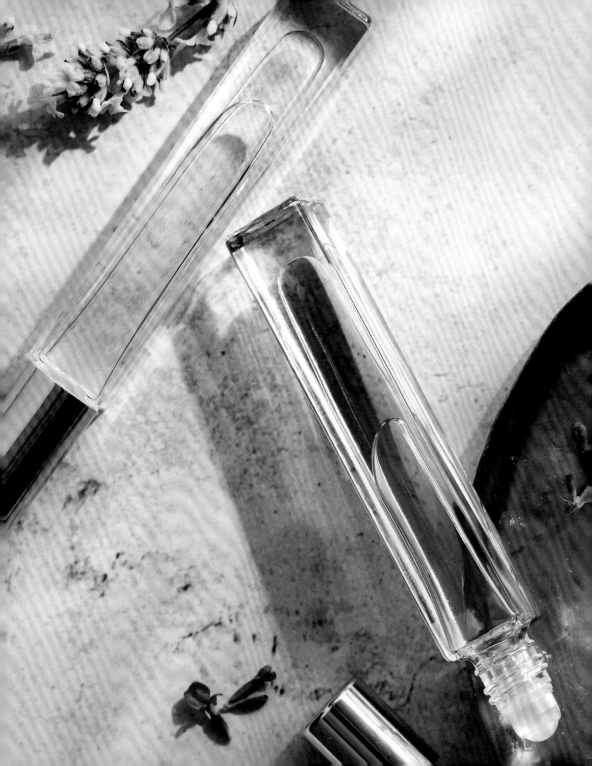

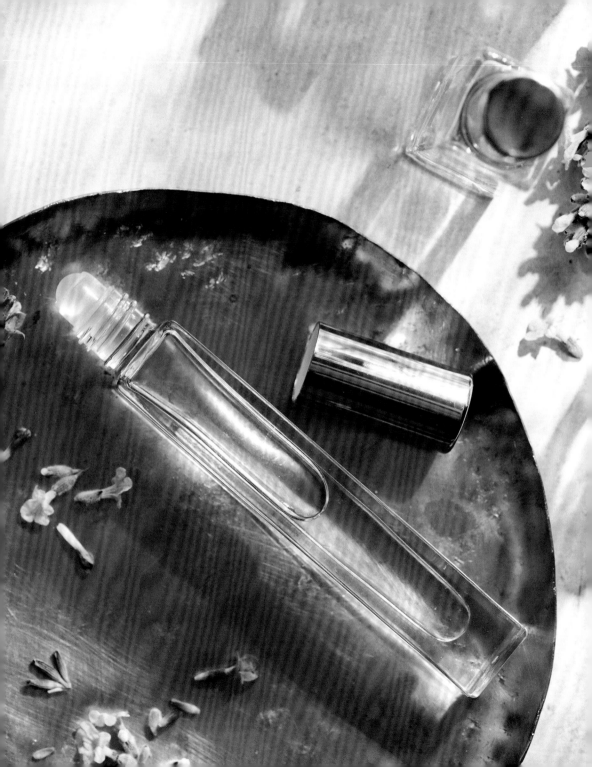

Eye of the Storm Roll-On Blend

These essential oils hold calming, uplifting, focusing, and grounding components. When a blend is right for you, its harmony is unmistakable. It's a scent you'll want to breathe in as deeply as your lungs will allow. Fresh and calming, this blend—along with some deep breathing—can help you find your own peaceful place in turbulent times.

1 (10-milliliter) glass roll-on bottle

7 drops black spruce essential oil

4 drops ho wood (*Cinnamomum camphora* var. linalool) essential oil

2 drops *L. angustifolia* lavender essential oil

2 drops frankincense essential oil

2 drops blue tansy (*Tanacetum annuum*) essential oil

1 drop ylang-ylang essential oil

2 teaspoons fractionated coconut oil

MAKES ABOUT 20 APPLICATIONS

• In the bottle, combine the essential oils, swirling gently to blend.

• Add the coconut oil, cap tightly, and shake to mix.

• Store in a cool, dark place. Keep out of reach of children.

TO USE: In a circular motion, apply to the sides of the neck and the pulse point on each wrist. Inhale deeply. Apply up to 3 times a day as needed. A note of caution: blue tansy oil can interact with drugs metabolized by CYP2D6 (such as beta-blockers, SSRIs, opiates, and others).

Blue Day Roll Away

Whether you're dragging your feet on a Monday morning or wishing winter would end, dab on this warm, aromatic blend of uplifting essences, and then take some cleansing breaths to elevate your mood and boost your spirit. The oils synergize together beautifully to help raise emotional lows and to smooth out the stressful bumps of the day.

1 (10-milliliter) glass roll-on bottle

3 drops *L. angustifolia* lavender essential oil

3 drops rose geranium essential oil

3 drops bergamot FCF (furocoumarin-free) essential oil

3 drops ylang-ylang essential oil

2 drops sweet orange essential oil

2 drops frankincense essential oil

1 drop holy basil (tulsi) essential oil

1 drop jasmine (*Jasminum grandiflorum*) absolute

2 teaspoons fractionated coconut oil

MAKES ABOUT 20 APPLICATIONS

◆ In the bottle, combine the essential oils and jasmine absolute, swirling gently to blend.

◆ Add the coconut oil, cap tightly, and shake to mix.

◆ Store in a cool, dark place. Keep out of reach of children.

TO USE: In a circular motion, apply to the sides of the neck and the pulse point on each wrist. Inhale deeply. Apply up to 3 times a day.

Sweet Dreams Diffuser Oil

Feel yourself drift away as this dreamy blend of essential oils soothes you to sleep—one deep, relaxing breath at a time.

3 drops *L. angustifolia* lavender essential oil

2 drops frankincense essential oil

1 drop ylang-ylang essential oil

1 drop Roman chamomile essential oil

MAKES 1 USE

TO USE: Add the essential oils to an aromatherapy diffuser. Sweet dreams!

Relaxing Bath Powder

For softening your skin, your mood, and your tensions, nothing beats a warm bath with this blend of oils that each hold naturally soothing components.

9 drops *L. angustifolia* lavender essential oil

6 drops Roman chamomile essential oil

3 drops ylang-ylang essential oil

6 tablespoons Natrasorb Bath, or 1 tablespoon carrier oil

1 (4-ounce) glass jar with airtight lid

MAKES ENOUGH FOR 3 USES

◆ In a small bowl, combine the essential oils. Swirl gently to blend.

◆ Add the Natrasorb to the bowl and use a fork to blend well.

◆ Transfer the mixture to the jar and cover tightly.

◆ Store in a cool, dark place. Keep out of reach of children.

TO USE: Fill a bathtub with water. Stir 2 tablespoons of the mixture into the water before entering the tub. Relax for 15 to 20 minutes. Rinse with fresh water and pat dry.

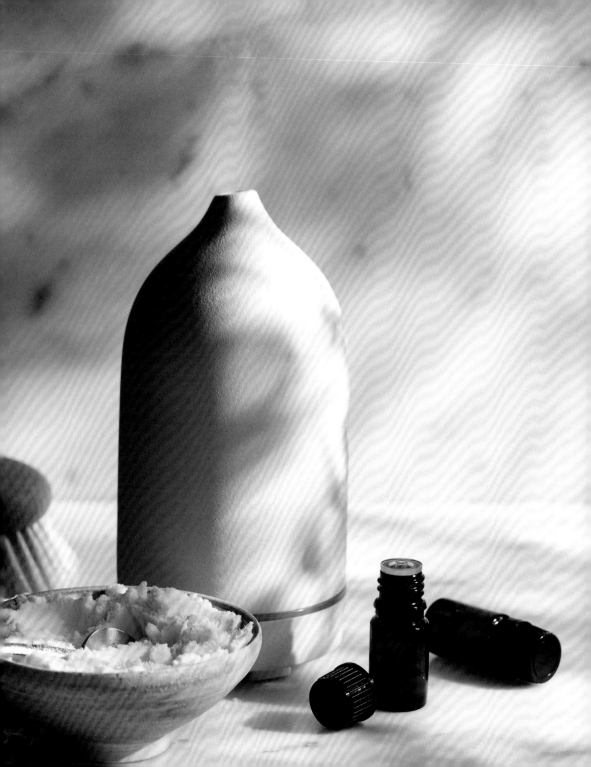

Skin

Your skin is a complex, ever-changing, living environment. And as unappealing as it may sound, the landscape of your skin is fully colonized by dense populations of vital microbial communities. In healthy skin, these bacteria, fungi, and even viruses create a healthy barrier to block invading pathogens.[1] You need this flora, this balanced ecosystem, the same way you need symbiotic bacteria in your gut. Lavender can help with this balance and much more.

ANTI-MICROBIAL SUPPORT

Some populations of microorganisms that live on your skin can shift from harmless to pathogenic if they aren't kept in check by other residents of the colony. Methicillin-resistant *Staphylococcus aureus* (MRSA) is a good example of one that's quick to overpopulate if given the slightest chance. The antimicrobial properties of diluted lavender oil can help with population control and keeping that delicate, healthy balance.[2] Emerging research has produced hopeful results in a test where lavender oil was effective against antibiotic-resistant superbugs such as MRSA (and *Escherichia coli*).[3] This is an exceptional quality for skin care, and one that can't be replicated in synthetic fragrances.

ANTIOXIDANT PROTECTION

Also prized in skin care are the antioxidant properties richly available in lavender essential oil.[4] These radical-scavenging properties are known to promote cell and tissue regeneration and combat the oxidative stress that ages skin before its time.

Quick & Easy Lavender Body Products

Want to enjoy the scent of lavender but don't have lots of free hours for projects? You can still whip up some lavender goodies in no time. Unscented base products—hand soap, shampoo, moisturizing lotion—can be purchased ready to customize and use by simply adding your own natural ingredients, such as lavender essential oil. (See Resources on page 187 for recommended suppliers.) These make great gifts too!

Follow the chart below, or to experiment, start with a drop of *L. angustifolia* lavender oil for each ounce of base product. Mix the lavender oil into the base and take a whiff. Repeat as needed to reach the desired fragrance strength.

BASE PRODUCT	NUMBER OF DROPS PER 1 CUP OF BASE
Lavender liquid hand soap	10 to 15
Lavender body wash	20 to 30
Lavender shampoo	20 to 30
Lavender lotion	10 to 20

• In an 8-ounce bottle or dispenser, add the drops of lavender essential oil according to the table above. Fill the bottle with about 1 cup of unscented liquid base, leaving 1 inch of headspace for mixing. Cap the bottle and shake gently to blend. If you're using a thick lotion, stir the mixture to blend (a chopstick works well). For shelf-life guidelines, see How to Store Lavender Oil on page 55.

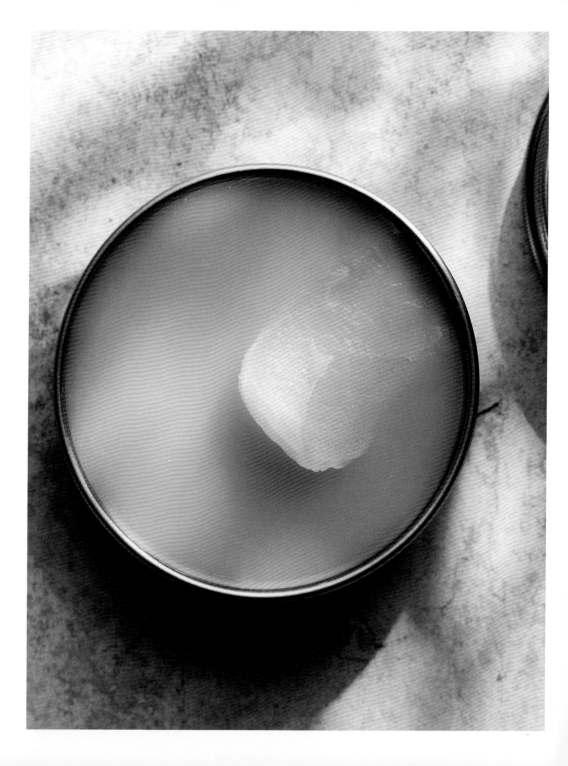

Lavender-Vanilla Lip Balm

If there's a perfect spot to enjoy the delicious aroma of pure vanilla and calming lavender, it's right under your nose. Relax, seal in moisture, and protect your lips all at the same time. A tin of homemade lip balm makes a memorable gift topper too.

1 tablespoon mango seed (*Mangifera indica*) butter

2 teaspoons ethically harvested, filtered organic beeswax pellets

2 teaspoons virgin (unrefined) coconut oil

¼ teaspoon jojoba oil

5 drops *L. angustifolia* lavender essential oil

1 drop vanilla absolute or vanilla CO_2 extract

1 (1-ounce) flat metal tin, glass container, or 5 lip balm tubes

MAKES 1 OUNCE

◆ Before you begin, review the Wax-Melting Safety Tips on page 67. In the top of a double boiler over medium heat, melt together the mango seed butter, beeswax, coconut oil, and jojoba oil. (Alternatively, melt the ingredients in a clean metal can or pitcher set into a pan of simmering water.)

◆ Remove from heat and mix in the lavender and vanilla.

◆ Transfer to the container. Cover and allow to harden, 4 to 8 hours.

TO USE: Apply to lips as desired.

Moisture-Locking Body Cream

Rough patches of skin will get a chance to heal when you protect them from moisture loss and also arm them with the antioxidants in this natural and lusciously scented cream.

2 tablespoons cocoa butter

2 tablespoons virgin (unrefined) coconut oil

4 tablespoons sweet almond oil

4 teaspoons arrowroot powder

24 drops *L. angustifolia* lavender essential oil

14 drops vanilla absolute or vanilla CO_2 extract

1 (4-ounce) glass jar with lid

MAKES 4 OUNCES

• In the top of a double boiler over medium heat, melt the cocoa butter and coconut oil together. (Alternatively, melt the ingredients in a clean metal can or pitcher set into a pan of simmering water.) Remove from heat.

• Add the sweet almond oil and arrowroot powder. Whisk together until smooth.

• Cover and refrigerate for 30 to 60 minutes, until the mixture becomes semisolid.

• Remove from the refrigerator. Whisk again until the mixture is creamy and white.

• Add the lavender and vanilla. Whisk a final time and transfer to the jar.

TO USE: Apply sparingly to patches of extra-dry skin as needed. Note that any oils that block moisture loss, such as cocoa butter and coconut oil, are comedogenic as well, meaning that extended use may clog pores.

Jasmine-Lavender Essential Perfume Oil

Night-blooming jasmine, lavender, and ylang-ylang mingle with warm wood and spicy pepper at the edge of the garden to bring you a joyful, natural fragrance that lasts for hours.

MAKES ABOUT 20 APPLICATIONS

1 (10-milliliter) glass roll-on bottle, or 2 (5-milliliter) roll-on bottles

14 drops sandalwood essential oil

6 drops lavender essential oil

2 drops ylang-ylang essential oil

2 drops black pepper essential oil

10 drops jasmine sambac (*Jasminum sambac*) absolute

2 teaspoons fractionated coconut oil

* In the bottle, combine the essential oils and jasmine sambac absolute, swirling gently to blend.

* Add the coconut oil, cap tightly, and shake to mix.

* Store in a cool, dark place. Keep out of reach of children.

TO USE: Apply a touch of this lingering fragrance onto the pulse points of your wrists or neck. Reapply as desired.

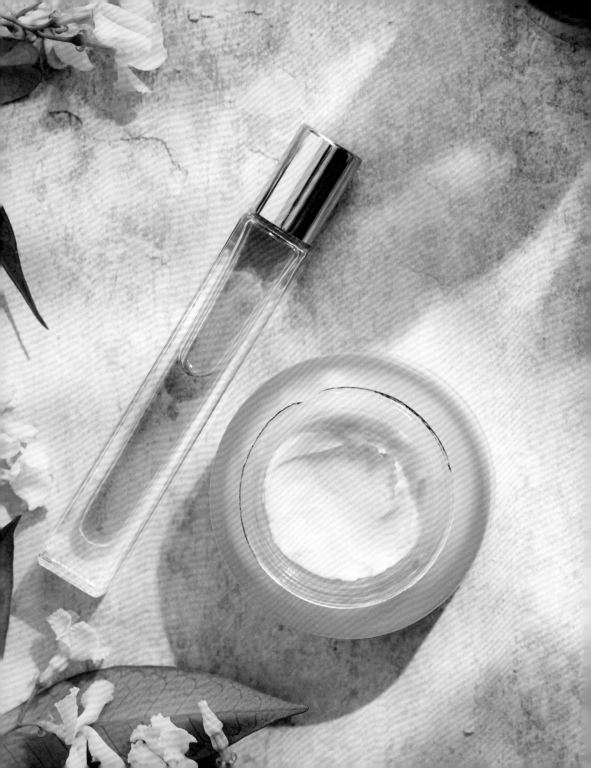

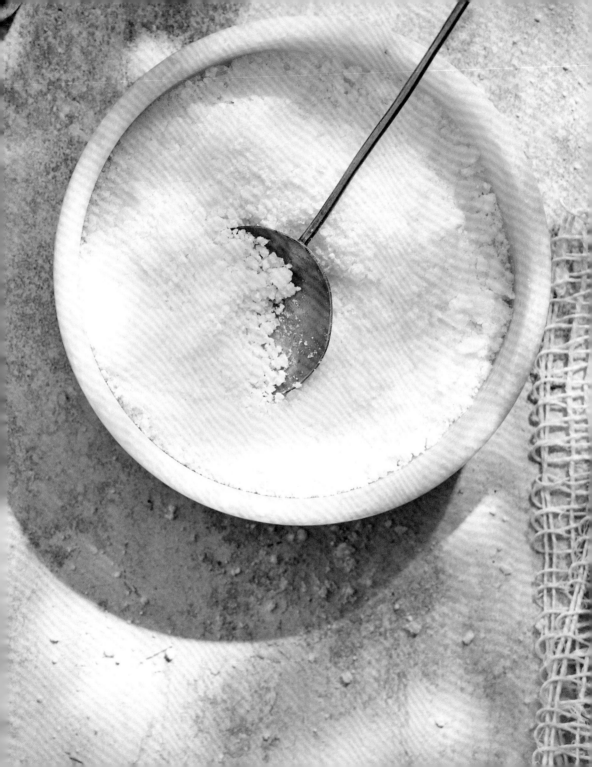

Antioxidant Steam Facial

When laden with the oils of lavender and green tea leaves, a cloud of steam will deliver antioxidants, help promote circulation, and soften blackheads for gentle extraction.

1 quart boiling water

1 tablespoon green tea leaves

2 to 3 drops *L. angustifolia* lavender essential oil

MAKES 1 FACIAL TREATMENT

TO USE: Into a large heatproof bowl, pour the boiling water. Add the tea leaves and lavender oil to the hot water. Be careful to approach steam slowly as you lean over the bowl. Cover your head and the bowl with a towel. Close your eyes to prevent irritation. Breathe deeply and allow the lavender to relax you while the fragrant steam does its work. Pull away for fresh air anytime the steam feels too hot, or if you feel light-headed. Continue treatment for about 5 minutes. Gently rinse face, pat dry, and moisturize.

Lavender & Rose Fizzy Bath Salts

Indulge in an exquisite floral bath, or treat a friend to a jar of these sparkling bath salts. The fragrance and silky feel of your bathwater will leave you feeling soothed and relaxed.

2/3 cup USP-approved Epsom salt

6 tablespoons baking soda

1/4 cup citric acid

3 tablespoons powdered whole milk, powdered goat milk, or organic coconut cream powder

2 1/2 tablespoons Natrasorb Bath

19 drops *L. angustifolia* lavender essential oil

4 drops rose absolute

1 (12-ounce) or 3 (4-ounce) glass jar(s) with airtight lid(s)

MAKES ENOUGH FOR 3 BATHS

• In a small bowl, mix together the Epsom salt, baking soda, citric acid, and powdered milk. Set aside.

• In a medium-sized bowl, use a fork to blend the Natrasorb with the essential oils and rose absolute.

• Add the Epsom salt mixture to the Natrasorb mixture and mix thoroughly.

• Transfer to the jar and store in a cool, dark place. Keep out of reach of children.

TO USE: Fill a bathtub with warm water. Pour 1/2 cup of bath salts into the water, and watch the fizzing action begin. Indulge in a leisurely soak for 15 to 20 minutes, and then rinse with fresh water.

Soothing Body Tea

To quiet your skin and your worries at the same time, brew a fragrant bath of dried botanicals. Ease into the tub and soak in these soothing and anti-inflammatory flowering herbs. For gift-giving, fill a 1-pint mason jar with herbs and include a few organza or muslin bags in the package, or fill a 1½-quart jar with individual bags of bathing herbs.

1½ cups dried lavender buds (*L. angustifolia* or lavandin)

¾ cup dried chamomile flowers

¾ cup dried rosebuds and/or petals

½ cup dried jasmine flowers

8 (3-by-4-inch) muslin, organza, or disposable drawstring tea bags

MAKES 8 SINGLE-USE BAGS

• In a large bowl, gently hand mix the dried flowers.

• Fill each muslin bag with ¼ cup of the mixed flowers. Pull the drawstrings tightly and tie with a bow.

• Store the bags in an airtight container.

TO USE: Fill a bathtub ¼ full with very hot water. Steep 1 bag of herbs in the hot bathwater for 5 minutes. Continue filling the tub to a comfortable temperature. Soak in the tub for about 20 minutes. Let the herbal bag float freely, and give it a squeeze every few minutes. When finished, empty and rinse the muslin bag. Hang to dry for another use.

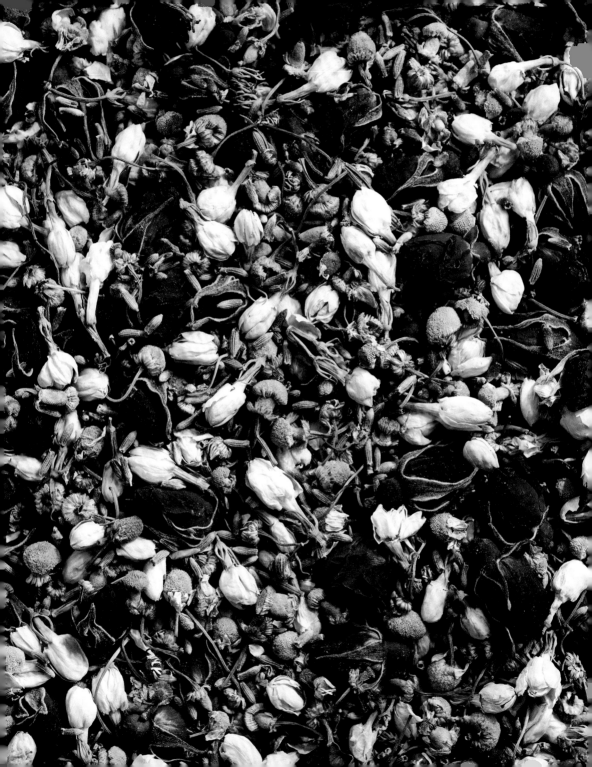

Home

Behind the clean scent of lavender is a hardworking crew of bioactive agents. Although this crew works to control specific pests, fungi, and germs, the greatest power of lavender essential oil lies in its ability to balance other oils and create even more potent synergy. When the goal is aggressive treatment of bacteria and fungi, blending lavender oil with specific essential oils can increase the joined antimicrobial effect.

In contrast, using corrosive, carcinogenic, or strongly irritating chemicals can certainly destroy germs and odors in the home, but over time those hostile chemicals can also be destructive to the health of people, pets, and our intricately connected environment. The Environmental Protection Agency (EPA) suggests using products that support the long-term well-being of people and the planet and offers common-sense guidelines to follow.[1] While even natural chemical compounds can harm our air, water, and health if they reach toxic quantities, by using pure essential oils to make your own home products you will tick these critical EPA boxes: biodegradable, noncarcinogenic, free of ozone-depleting substances, produced from renewable resources, and minimally, reusably packaged.

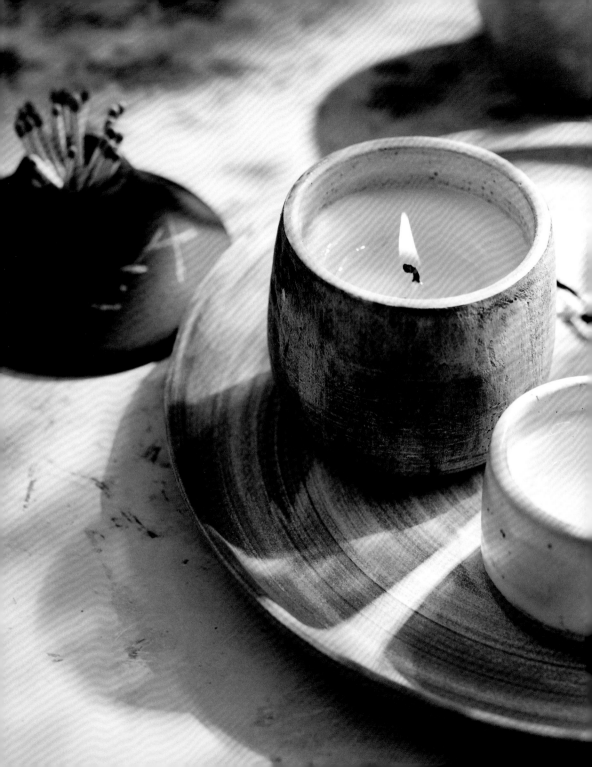

Lavender Beeswax Candle

A relaxing lavender ambience can be even more special when you make your own candles with pure essential oil and sustainable wax, free of artificial chemicals or colors. Research shows that beeswax candles burn longer and cleaner than paraffin or soy wax.[2]

Wick sticker (optional)
1 (4-ounce) heatproof glass jar, or multiple smaller heatproof containers
Medium cotton wick with metal tab attached
Wick-centering tool or wooden clothespin
3¼ ounces (about 10½ tablespoons) ethically harvested, filtered organic beeswax pellets
1½ teaspoons lavandin essential oil

MAKES 1 CANDLE

◆ Adhere the wick sticker to the center of the jar bottom. Press the wick's metal tab over the sticker to attach the wick. Or use a bit of melted wax to secure the wick to the bottom and let the wax harden for 10 minutes before filling the jar with wax.

◆ Center the top of the wick. A burning wick that is off-center can cause the glass to break. There are a lot of ways to keep the wick centered (see photo #1 on page 104). Most candle-making kits come with a centering tool, but you might find a clothespin to be the simplest solution.

◆ Review the Wax-Melting Safety Tips on page 67. In the bottom of a double boiler, heat about 1 inch of water. Add wax pellets to the top of the double boiler and set over the water. (Alternatively, melt the ingredients in a clean metal can or pitcher set into a pan of simmering water. A disposable can will save on cleanup time!)

Note: If you'd like to make multiple candles, purchase 1 pound of wax to fill 5 (4-ounce) jars.

◆ Over medium-low heat, melt the wax. Use a cooking thermometer to check the temperature of the wax and keep it at 160 to 170 degrees F. Add water to refill the bottom pan as needed. Do not let the wax temperature exceed 180 degrees F. Check often. The wax should melt completely within 10 to 20 minutes.

$\longrightarrow$

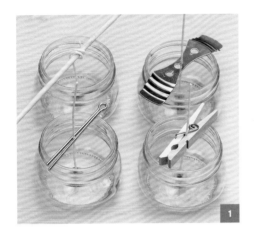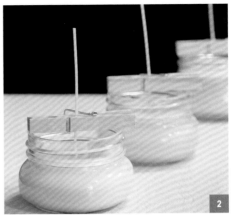

• When the wax is fully melted, add the lavender. Stir gently until blended. (A disposable chopstick works nicely!)

• Cool the wax to about 155 degrees F, and *slowly* pour it into the jar. Leave ½ inch of headspace. (See photo #2, above.)

• In a warm place, let cool for 1 hour.

• Top off with more melted wax if needed to fill cracks or sinkholes. Allow the wax to fully harden in a warm area for at least 24 hours.

TO USE: Fragrance emerges not from the wick, but from a melted pool of wax, so before each use trim the wick to ¼ inch (nail clippers work well for this). On the first lighting, it's important to let the candle burn long enough to melt the entire top surface of wax to prevent tunneling. This takes about an hour per inch of candle width, so burn a 2-inch-wide candle for at least 2 hours.

Lavender-Scented Hand Sanitizer

While nothing works better than a proper soap-and-water cleansing, hand sanitizer can help fight germs when you don't have access to a sink. Lavender itself is not an antiviral agent, but it will add fragrance and some antibacterial and antifungal properties to a true disinfectant. According to the guidelines offered by the Centers for Disease Control and Prevention (CDC), an effective sanitizer made with rubbing alcohol must contain at least 70 percent isopropanol. So if your homemade formula is diluted with skin softener and fragrance, you need to start with rubbing alcohol that is 99 percent isopropanol, and be careful to ensure that the rubbing alcohol makes up at least 71 percent of the total ingredients.

¾ cup 99 percent isopropyl alcohol
¼ cup aloe vera gel
8 to 10 drops lavandin essential oil
1 (8-ounce) sterilized glass or PET plastic bottle with leakproof top or pump dispenser

MAKES 8 OUNCES

• Sterilize a large glass container and spoon. If the container does not have a spout, sterilize a funnel too.

• Without touching the ingredients with your hands, add them all to the container. Stir with the spoon to mix.

• Transfer to the bottle and cap tightly.

• Let sanitizer rest for 72 hours before use.

Yoga Mat Freshening Mist

For a fresh citrus and lavender scent, and to discourage fungal and microbial activity on your yoga mat, gym mat, or weight bench, simply spritz this mist on your exercise surfaces. (Note that this is not an antiviral sanitizer.)

1 (4-ounce) amber or cobalt glass bottle with sprayer
2 tablespoons white distilled vinegar or witch hazel
20 drops lemon essential oil
20 drops *L. angustifolia* lavender essential oil
20 drops sweet orange essential oil
Up to 6 tablespoons distilled water

MAKES 4 OUNCES

♦ In the spray bottle, combine the vinegar and essential oils. Swirl gently to blend.

♦ Add the distilled water slowly to fill the bottle. Cap tightly and shake well.

♦ Store in a cool, dark place. Keep out of reach of children.

TO USE: Shake the bottle before each use. Lightly spray yoga mat or equipment. Wipe down if desired.

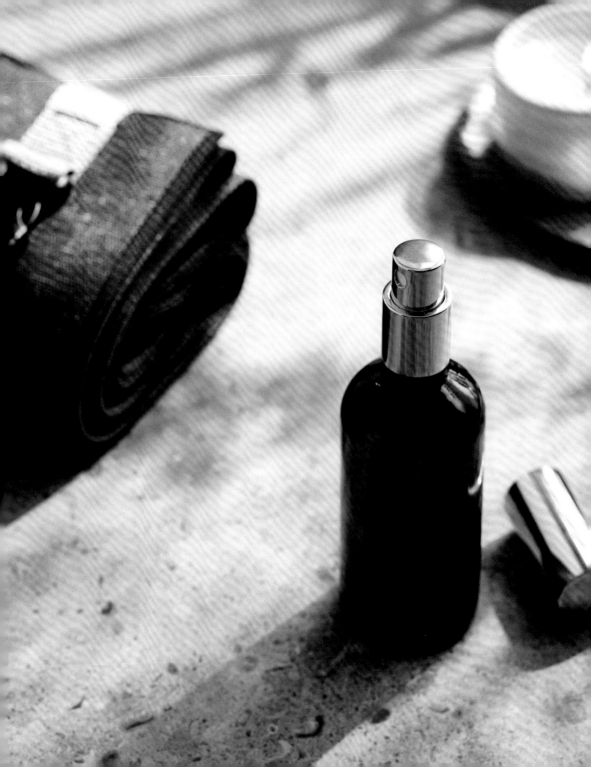

Sunshine Air Freshener

Wherever odors linger, you can quickly spruce up the air with the fresh, calming aroma of this floral blend.

1 (4-ounce) amber or cobalt glass bottle with sprayer

2 tablespoons 160-proof vodka

42 drops lavandin essential oil

24 drops geranium essential oil

12 drops ylang-ylang essential oil

12 drops ho wood (*Cinnamomum camphora* var. linalool) essential oil

6 tablespoons distilled water

MAKES 4 OUNCES

◆ In the spray bottle, combine the vodka and essential oils. Swirl gently to blend.

◆ Slowly add the distilled water, cap tightly, and shake well.

◆ Store in a cool, dark place. Keep out of reach of children.

TO USE: Shake bottle before each use. Spritz the air as desired.

Vacuum Breeze

Fill your home with fresh, natural scents every time you run the vacuum.

1 cotton ball or 100 percent wool felt ball

2 drops lavandin essential oil

2 drops pine or Douglas fir essential oil

1 drop lemon essential oil

MAKES 1 BALL

◆ To avoid skin contact, use gloves or tweezers to hold the cotton ball.

◆ Drop the essential oils onto the ball.

TO USE: Place the ball into the vacuum canister or bag. Replace as desired. Keep out of reach of children.

Lavender Leaves

Lavender flowers catch the eye. And though the flowers contain more and higher-quality essential oil than other parts of the lavender plant, the often-discarded leaves of lavender have practical uses too.

Crush a lavender leaf between your fingers. The fragrance is unmistakably lavender, with a slightly sharper note. A recent test in Poland showed that while *L. angustifolia* leaves held some sought-after linalool and linalyl acetate, the harsher components such as camphor, eucalyptol, and borneol were dominant. Interestingly though, when lavender leaves were convection dried at 140 degrees F, the ratio of sweet to sharp components changed.[3] The drying of leaves under the right conditions altered the flavor profile so dramatically that dried lavender leaves could be used in cooking much the same way as rosemary.

Fresh or dried, you can also use lavender leaves to make floral water for a pillow spray, ironing spray, or even to concoct a monster-under-the-bed banishing spray.

LAVENDER LEAF WATER

¼ cup crushed or chopped lavender leaves (dried or fresh)
Small muslin drawstring bag
1¼ cups water

MAKES 1 CUP

+ Scoop the lavender leaves into a reusable muslin bag. Tie the drawstrings.

+ In a small pan, bring the water to a boil. Remove from heat.

+ Add the tied bag of lavender leaves. Cover and steep overnight.

+ Squeeze and remove the bag. Pour the scented water into an 8-ounce spray bottle and use as desired.

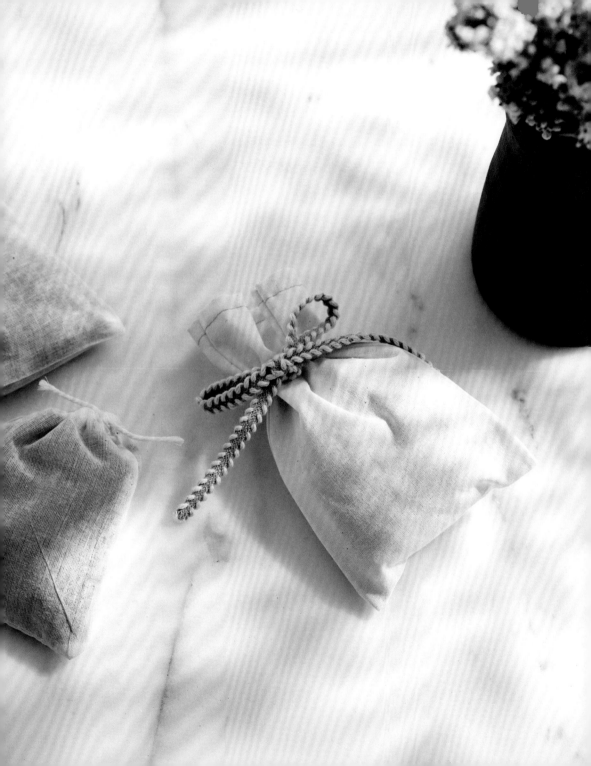

Lavender Bags for Dryers & Drawers

Place these refreshers, filled with nature's deodorizing herbs, in shoes, drawers, cabinets, closets, cars, beds, and backpacks—wherever you want the clean fragrance of lavender. Or freshen your laundry without synthetic chemicals: just squeeze and toss a bag into the dryer. Although the aroma of the lavender pouch is strong, only a wispy fragrance will remain on your clothing.

To make an environmentally chic gift kit, place a handcrafted refresher, some replacement pouches, and a small bottle of lavandin essential oil into a basket. This pure-green gift keeps on giving naturally lavender-scented laundry for up to a full year.

3 cups (3 to 4 ounces) lavandin buds
2 tablespoons minced dried orange peel (optional)
18 whole cloves (optional)
6 (3-by-4-inch) natural muslin drawstring bags
1 (12½-by-6½-inch) piece of natural-fiber fabric
Color-coordinated thread
18 inches of ¼- to ⅜-inch-wide washable trim or grosgrain ribbon
Clear, waterproof glue or Dritz Fray Check
Tools for Sewing Projects (page 119)

MAKES 1 BAG AND 6 INNER POUCHES

◆ Combine the lavandin and orange peel in a medium bowl.

◆ For the inner pouches, add ½ cup of the lavandin mixture plus 3 cloves to each muslin bag. Pull the drawstrings tightly so no buds can escape. Knot the strings and snip off the ends. (See photo #1 on page 112.)

◆ For the exterior bag, lay the fabric on the ironing board, right side down. Fold the short edges of the fabric toward you ⅜ inch. Press. Fold again ½ inch and press the double fold in place. Stitch the double-fold hem ¼ inch from the edge. (See photo #2 on page 112.)

◆ Return the fabric to the ironing board, right side down. Fold the long edges of the fabric toward you ⅜ inch. Press. Fold again ½ inch, and press the double fold in place. (See photo #3 on page 112.)

$\longrightarrow$

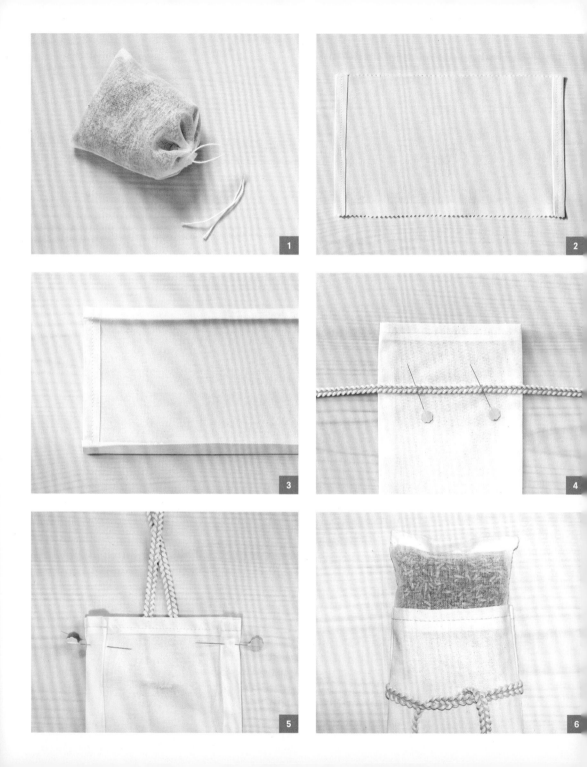

- Turn the fabric right side up. Place the middle of the ribbon in the center of the fabric, 1½ inches from one hemmed edge. Pin in place.

- At the center point, sew the ribbon to the fabric with a few stitches. Reinforce the stitching. (See photo #4, opposite.)

- Fold the fabric in half, right sides together, matching up the hemmed edges. Pin as needed to secure the double folds. (See photo #5, opposite.)

- Stitch the sides with a ⅜-inch seam allowance.

- Turn right side out. Push out the corners to square them (a chopstick is great for this), and press the bag flat.

- Insert a lavender-filled pouch. Wrap the ends of the ribbon around the bag and tie a knot. (See photo #6, opposite.) To keep the ribbon from fraying, cleanly trim ends at an angle. Apply a dab of clear waterproof glue to each angled cut.

TO USE: Squeeze the bag to release a fresh array of essential oil fragrance, and then toss it into the dryer with clothes. To extend the life span of the scent, store in an airtight container between uses. When the scent begins to fade, you can refresh the inner pouch with 2 to 3 drops of lavandin oil, or replace the pouch and use the old one in a drawer or laundry hamper.

Note: For use as a laundry refresher, the outer bag is needed to protect clothing from essential oil stains and to protect the lightweight inner pouch from breaking open in the dryer. For use as a deodorizing refresher, the inner pouch can be used with or without the outer bag.

Give

When your gift is handmade using the oils or flowers of lavender, you're sharing the goodness of lavender as well as showing your love. And you'll benefit too, because not only is handcrafting with lavender a delightful antidote for stress, but the act of giving itself can boost well-being.

Researchers have noted that when people sacrifice time or money to help others, the giver's brain releases dopamine—the feel-good neurotransmitter. The givers also reported a stronger feeling of well-being from altruistic giving than from spending time or money on personal pleasure.[1]

Another study explored how giving can strengthen relationships. Positive relationships foster emotional health, which in turn helps support the immune system. The study revealed that the recipient of a gift feels a stronger connection to the giver when the gift is an experience they will remember.[2]

So, how can you reap wellness benefits from giving gifts that forge stronger relationships? Try giving a lavender experience made with your own hands!

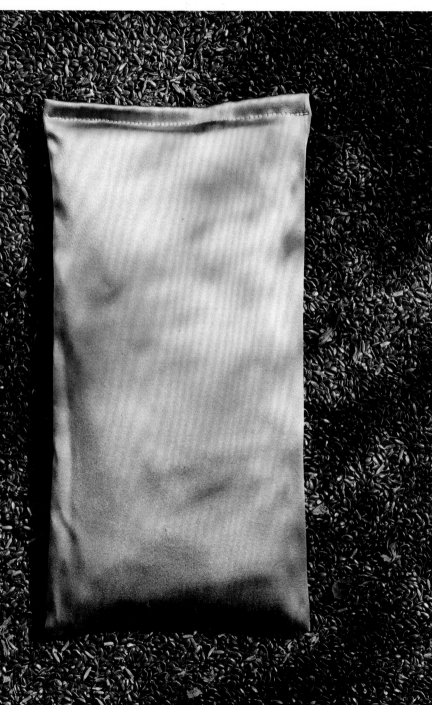

Soothing Eye Pillow

Mix the calmness of lavender, the coolness of peppermint, and the comforting weight of flaxseeds into this eye pillow that can be frozen for cool relief or microwaved for moist warmth. Choose whatever lavender variety calls to you and calms you. Lavandin buds offer some relaxing benefits plus a stronger, longer-lasting fragrance, and they are preferred by many over the softer-scented but more calming *L. angustifolia* buds.

1½ cups flaxseed (about 9 ounces) or rice (if allergic to flaxseed)

2 tablespoons dried lavender buds (*L. angustifolia* or lavandin)

2 tablespoons crushed dried peppermint leaves

2 (6-by-11-inch) pieces of soft, natural-fiber fabric

Color-coordinated cotton thread

Tools for Sewing Projects (page 119)

Note: If you don't have much sewing experience, avoid slippery material such as silk; choose high-quality cotton instead.

MAKES 1 (5-BY-10-INCH) EYE PILLOW

◆ In a large bowl, mix the flaxseed, lavender, and peppermint. Don't add any essential oils here as they can cause irritation to the eyes. Set aside. (See photo #1 on page 118.)

◆ Lay both pieces of fabric on the ironing board, right sides down. Press. Fold the top edges of each piece ½ inch toward the inside of the fabric. Press the folds. (See photo #2 on page 118.)

◆ Match up the top edges, right sides together, and pin as needed. (See photo #3 on page 118.)

◆ Stitch the sides and bottom with ½-inch seam allowance. Leave the top open. Clip the corners at an angle. (See photo #4 on page 118.)

◆ Turn right side out. Push out the corners to square them (a chopstick is great for this). Press. Topstitch around the sides and bottom, ⅛ inch from the edge. Be sure to start and stop stitching ⅛ inch from the top edge. (See photo #5 on page 118.)

⟶

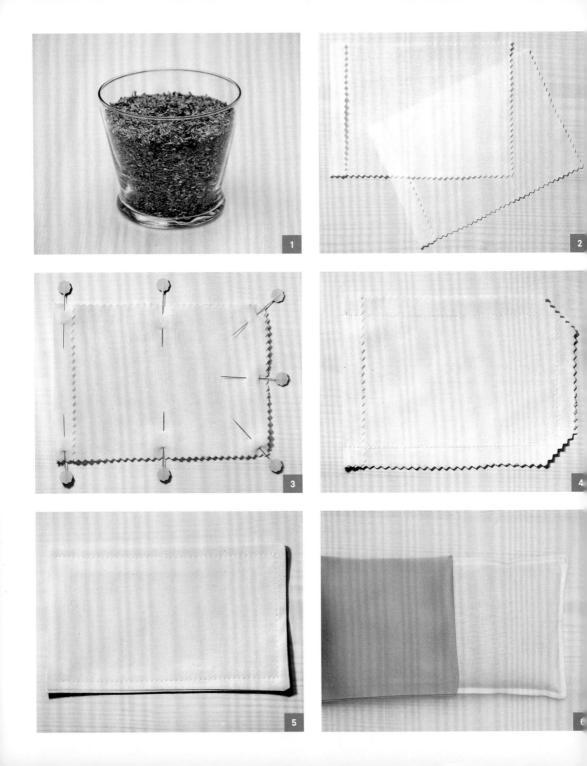

• Fill the fabric pouch with the flaxseed mixture, and shake the buds toward the bottom. Keeping the filling away from the needle, stitch the top closed with ⅛-inch topstitching. If desired, sew a washable cover (see Variation, below), and then slide the muslin pillow into it. (See photo #6, opposite.)

TO USE: To chill, enclose the eye pillow in a protective bag and freeze for at least an hour. To heat, microwave the pillow for 30 seconds. Shake to prevent hot spots and then microwave again for 15 seconds. Do not overheat!

Variation: For a silk pillow or a washable cover, follow the steps to sew an inner pillow of breathable muslin that will hold the herbs and protect the silk from oil that is released from the buds when heated. For the outer covering, you'll need 2 pieces of silk or prewashed fabric that are 6½ by 12 inches. Follow the steps on page 123 for making a cover.

Tools for Sewing Projects

• Sewing machine, including needles and basic attachments (or a hand-sewing needle and a lot of patience)
• Scissors
• Pinking shears (optional)
• Iron
• Ironing board or ironing mat
• Measuring tape (or a long ruler)
• Straight pins
• Seam ripper

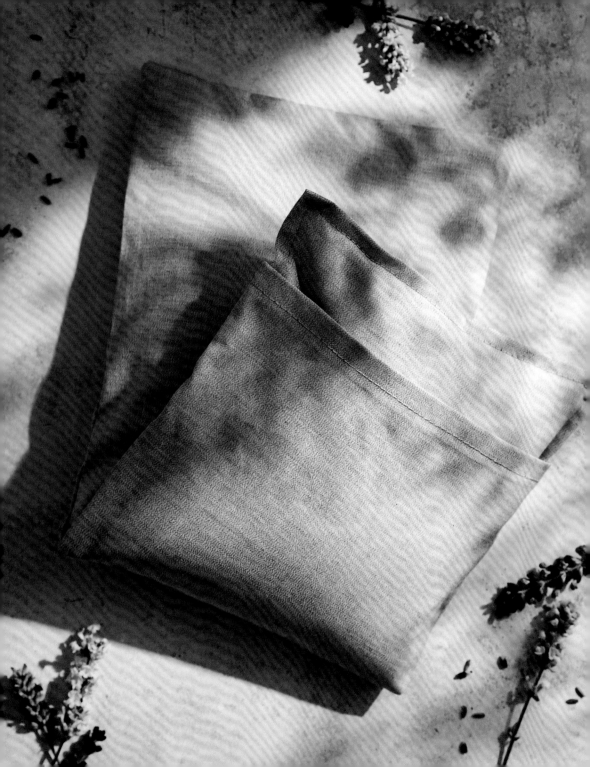

Aromatherapy Wrap with Washable Cover

The lavender fragrance of this wrap will bloom when microwaved, and the flaxseed filling will snuggle comfortably against any part of your body. Drape its therapeutic warmth around your neck, or chill the wrap to soothe inflamed joints. For personalized gifts, blend another favorite scent into the lavender filling.

For the wrap

6 cups flaxseed (about 2⅓ pounds) or rice (if allergic to flaxseed)
¼ cup dried lavandin buds
4 drops bergamot citrus essential oil or another favorite oil that blends with lavender
2 (8-by-17-inch) pieces of natural-fiber fabric
Color-coordinated cotton thread

For the cover

2 (8½-by-18½-inch) pieces of soft, pre-washed fabric
Color-coordinated thread

Tools for Sewing Projects (page 119)

MAKES 1 (7-BY-16-INCH) WRAP

◆ In a large bowl, mix the flaxseed, lavandin, and essential oil. Set aside.

◆ To make the wrap, lay both pieces of fabric on the ironing board right sides down. Press. Fold the top edges of each piece ½ inch toward the inside of the fabric. Press the folds. (See photo #2 on page 118.)

◆ Match up the top edges, right sides together, and pin as needed. (See photo #3 on page 118.)

◆ Stitch the sides and bottom with ½-inch seam allowance. Leave the top open. Clip the corners at an angle. (See photo #4 on page 118.)

◆ Turn right side out. Push out the corners to square them (a chopstick is great for this). Press. Topstitch around the sides and bottom, ⅛ inch from the edge. Be sure to start and stop stitching ⅛ inch from the top edge. (See photo #5 on page 118.)

◆ Fill the wrap with the flaxseed mixture, and shake the buds toward the bottom. Keeping the filling away from the needle, stitch the top closed with ⅛-inch topstitching. (See photo #6 on page 118.)

⟶

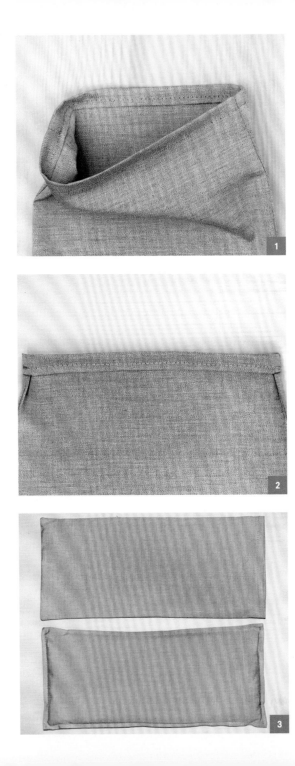

- To make the cover, begin by prewashing any fabric that shrinks when laundered, and then press the fabric right side down. Cut pieces to size.

- Lay the pieces of fabric on the ironing board, right sides down. Fold the top edges of each piece ½ inch toward the inside of the fabric. Press the folds. (See photo #2 on page 118.)

- Match up the top edges, right sides together, and pin as needed. (See photo #3 on page 118.)

- Stitch the sides and bottom with ½-inch seam allowance. Leave the top open. Clip the corners at an angle *only* if you don't plan to finish the edges with French seams. (See photo #4 on page 118.)

- If you clip the corners, then finish the raw edges with zig-zag stitching or a serger. If you want all of the raw edges hidden, finish them with French seams. (See photo #1, opposite.)

- Fold the top edges ⅜ inch toward the inside of the fabric. Press. Fold again ½ inch and press the double fold in place. Pin as needed and stitch the double-fold hem around the opening, ¼ inch from the edge. (See photo #2, opposite.)

- Turn right side out. Push out the corners to square them. Press as needed. (See photo #3, opposite.)

TO USE: For heat therapy, microwave the inner wrap for 30 seconds at a time, shaking up the filling after each heating cycle until the desired temperature is reached. Do not overheat! After heating, slide the inner wrap into its cover. If desired, add drops of lavender oil to the inner wrap to strengthen or refresh aroma as needed. For a cold compress, seal the wrap in a protective bag and freeze for at least 2 hours.

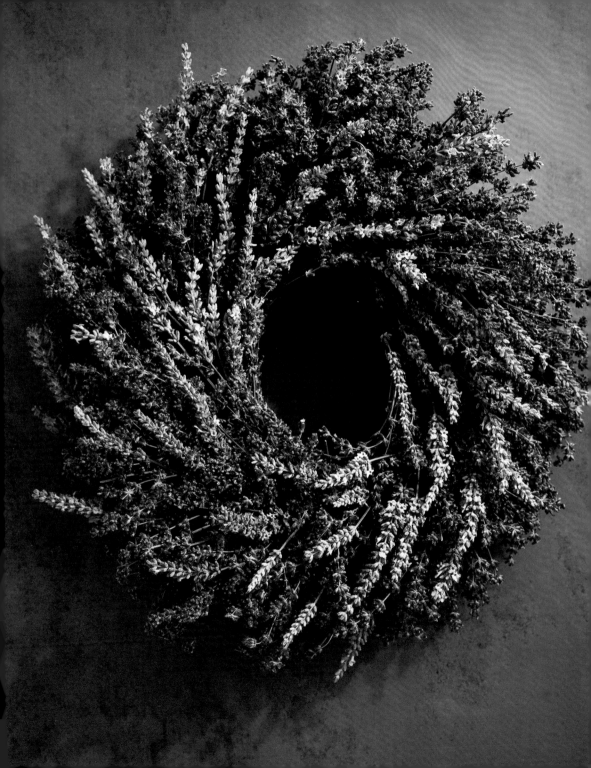

Twig & Lavender Wreath

Dangle the inviting fragrance of a lavender field over your front door, or create a memorable handmade gift. The frame for this wreath is made from the young shoot of a tree. When green and thin, these shoots are supple, and when dry, they hold their shape.

For best lavender results, harvest before the flowers open, and let the stalks dry for about a week. (If you use fully dried lavender, you'll lose a lot of buds while making the wreath.) You can also use freshly cut lavender if you check and retighten the wire a few times as the stems dry and shrink.

1 thin, pliable 5-foot-long shoot cut from a tree (leaves removed), or 1 premade round 8-inch grapevine wreath frame
8 to 16 bundles of partly dried lavender (about 100 stems each)
Spool of 20-to-24-gauge wire or natural twine
3 feet of wide ribbon (optional)

MAKES 1 WREATH

◆ Twist and weave the slender shoot into an 8-inch circle. Beginning with the thickest end of the shoot, wrap the thinner end around the circle, weaving it under and over the thicker ring. No tools or glue are needed, but you can use twine to secure any unruly spots until the frame hardens in place.

◆ Wrap wire twice around one point of the woven frame, and twist the wires together to secure it. This will be your starting point. Using wire instead of twine makes it easier to tighten any loose places later as lavender stems dry.

◆ Split the lavender bundles into bunches of 25 to 100 stems each. The more stems per bunch, the fuller the wreath will be.

◆ With scissors or hand pruners, trim each handful evenly, 6 to 8 inches in length, leaving a couple of inches of stem below the flower heads.

$\longrightarrow$

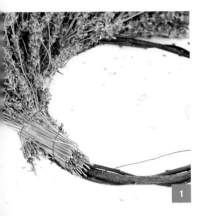

• Hold 1 bunch of lavender lengthwise against the wood frame. Wrap the wire tightly around the stems and frame a few times to secure the lavender to the frame. (See photo #1.)

• Repeat with each lavender bunch, working your way around the frame, checking each time that no gaps are visible from the front side.

• The final bundle takes extra maneuvering. Carefully lift up the flower heads of the first bundle that you attached. Push the stems of the final bundle underneath the raised flower heads. Wrap wire around the final bunch of stems without damaging the raised flowers. (See photo #2.)

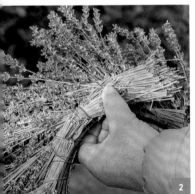

• Secure the wire and create a loop for hanging: Cut the wire with wire cutters, leaving an 8-inch tail of wire. Push the end of the tail under the last row of wire. Pull the tail snug and bend it into a loop. Push the end of the tail under the wire again, and twist it tightly around the wires.

• With scissors, closely trim any stems that jut out and prevent the wreath from resting evenly when hanging. (See photo #3.)

• To tighten loose wires as needed over time, use pliers to hold and twist any slack on the back side of the wreath.

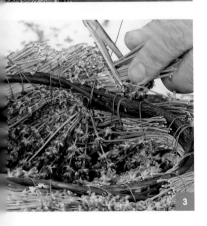

TO USE: Hang the wreath using the wire loop or with a wide ribbon. Have fun with accents! Tie on a big bow, wire in some pine cones, poke in some painted thistles, or weave in a few of your favorite dried botanicals.

Fragrant Lavender Fire Starter

Even the scraps of a lavender harvest can be useful. After stripping buds for fragrance and cooking, save those bare stalks in a shoebox or paper bag. Use individual stalks as grilling sticks or aromatic kindling, or bundle the stems together to make these fragrant, giftable fire starters.

6 ounces coconut wax or scrap wax from leftover candles

7 feet of natural twine

3 handfuls of lavender or lavandin stalks (500 to 600 total), stripped and trimmed to the same length

6 extra-long twist ties or standard rubber bands

3 (6-by-2½-inch) strips of paper (used bags or old gift wrap work great)

9 lavender stalks with buds (optional)

MAKES 3 FIRE STARTERS

◆ Chop the wax into small chunks as desired for quicker melting.

◆ Cut 3 (6-inch) pieces of twine for wicks. Cut the remaining twine into 3 equal pieces.

◆ Lay some parchment or waxed paper near the stove.

◆ Review the Wax-Melting Safety Tips on page 67. In the bottom pan of a double boiler, heat about 1 inch of water. Add the wax to the top of the double boiler and set over the water. (Alternatively, set a clean metal pitcher or can into a pan of simmering water and put the wax inside.)

◆ Over medium-low heat, melt the wax. Use a cooking thermometer to check the temperature of the wax, which should be kept below 150 degrees F. Add water as needed to refill the pan.

◆ While the wax is melting, divide the stems into 3 bundles.

◆ In the center of each bundle, lay a 6-inch piece of twine lengthwise with 1 inch of wick extending from the top of each bundle. Hold a bundle tightly with one hand. Evenly match up the ends.

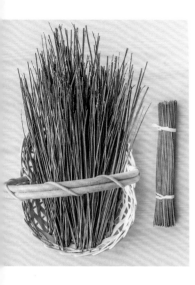

• Wrap extra-long twist ties or rubber bands tightly around the ends of each bundle, about an inch from the ends (see photo, left).

• Remove the fully melted wax from the heat, and let it cool to about 120 degrees F. The wax will become milky instead of clear. Dip an end of a bundle about ½ inch into the wax. (The wax should not reach the twist tie.) Raise and hold for 10 seconds, or until the dripping stops. If the wax does not stick to the ends, allow it to cool a little more, and then dip the bundle again.

• Snugly wrap a paper strip around the center of each bundle. Holding the paper in place, wrap twine around the paper several times and tie a knot. Carefully remove the twist ties. Repeat for all bundles.

• Scrape excess wax from the wicks. For gifting, slide a few lavender flowers into each paper sleeve.

TO USE: Place a lavender fire starter under some sticks and logs, leaving the wick accessible. Light and enjoy.

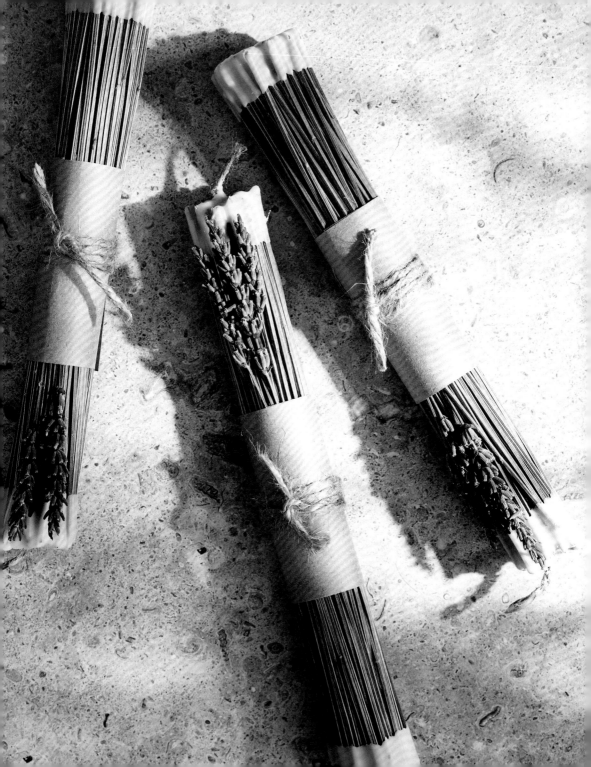

Taste

A colorful plant-forward diet—with a variety of fresh fruits, vegetables, and natural herbs such as lavender—holds a rich array of micronutrients. These vitamins, minerals, and phytonutrients are absorbed and put to work by your body to support your health.

Phytonutrients (literally translated as "plant nutrients") are also known as phytochemicals. Like vitamins and minerals, they are chemical compounds. When absorbed together, these compounds synergize in ways that are known to exist but are not yet fully understood. Thousands of phyto-nutrients are being studied from plants around the world, and the specific phytochemicals in lavender are being tested for potential antioxidant, cytotoxic, antibacterial, and preventative roles they may play in diet.

Your goal is not to eat a handful of lavender! A thimbleful of lavender will flavor an entire pot or punch bowl. In a teaspoon-sized serving of lavender, you'll get about 1 percent of the body's daily need for iron and even less of the micronutrients vitamin D, calcium, and potassium. But experts agree that a healthy diet should focus on variety and nutrient density, and in that way lavender can play a small but integral part in supporting your overall wellness and a healthy immune system.

CULINARY LAVENDER

"Culinary" or "food grade" lavender means that the lavender is a low-camphor variety, grown without chemicals or pesticides, and processed in a sanitary way that is safe to eat.

Varieties of *L. angustifolia*, with their mild and sweet fragrances, are preferred by most chefs, especially in sweet dishes. Other species can smell strongly of camphor, but lavandin has a couple of exceptions. The varieties 'Provence' and 'Super' are fairly mild in camphor, and used sparingly, they can flavor meats and savory dishes with an edgy floral bite. Even mild lavandins have a stronger taste than *L. angustifolia*, so if you're using lavandin, begin with half the quantity of *L. angustifolia* called for in the recipe—or your food could taste oddly akin to soap.

'Hidcote Blue'   'Buena Vista'   'Melissa'   'Betty's Blue'   'Folgate'   'Royal Velvet'   'Munstead'

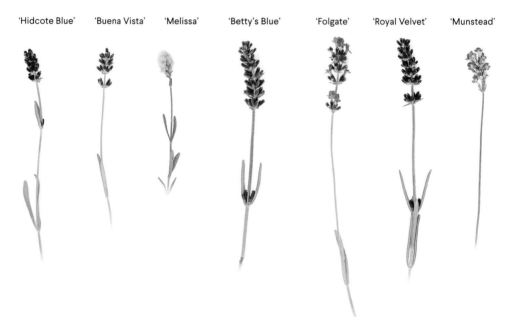

A few favorite culinary varieties of *L. angustifolia*. These flowers taste much the same as their fragrance—sweet and floral with a resonant minty impression.

Fresh & Dried Lavender Equivalents

Flavor increases as lavender flowers dry, and even more so when ground with a pestle or a spice grinder. To make substitutions in recipes, start with these guidelines and adjust for personal taste:

1 tablespoon fresh lavender = 1½ teaspoons dried lavender
1½ teaspoons dried lavender = ½ teaspoon ground lavender

The easiest way to grind dried lavender is in a spice grinder or coffee grinder. Simply pulse lavender buds for a few seconds at a time, stopping when the lavender is as coarse or fine in texture as you want. A mortar and pestle work well for bruising lavender buds to better release their fragrance, or to coarsely grind a small quantity of lavender buds.

FLAVORS THAT PAIR WITH LAVENDER

Lavender adds a sweet touch of herbal complexity to breads, soups, beverages, and creamy desserts. Assertive floral notes balance naturally with zesty top notes like lemon, ginger, and citrus, and with sharp flavors like balsamic vinegar, goat cheese, and smoked meats. One way to experiment is to substitute lavender for its closest culinary cousin, rosemary, in your favorite savory recipe.

Lavender Flavor Pairings

Fruits	Apricot, blackberry, blueberry, cantaloupe, cherry, coconut, cranberry, fig, grape, grapefruit, honeydew, kiwi, lemon, lime, nectarine, orange, peach, pear, pineapple, plum, pomegranate, raspberry, strawberry, tangerine
Vegetables	Beet, carrot, cucumber, mushroom, onion, potato, pumpkin, sweet potato, tomato
Grains	Cornmeal, oats, pasta, rice
Milks & Creams	Buttermilk, cream, ice cream, yogurt
Cheeses	Mild (cream cheese, fontina, mascarpone, Monterey Jack, mozzarella, ricotta), strong (blue, Brie, feta, goat, Gorgonzola, Parmesan)
Meats	Chicken, lamb, pork, salmon, smoked fish, turkey
Nuts	Almonds, cashews, pecans, walnuts
Legumes	Lentils, white beans
Savory Pastries	Biscuits, breads, cornbread, scones
Desserts	Brownies, cakes, chocolates, cookies, cream pies, fruit cobblers
Sweeteners	Agave syrup, honey, maple syrup, molasses, sugar
Alcohols	Apple brandy, gin, rosé, vodka, whiskey
Juices	Apple cider, ginger ale, lemonade
Teas	Chamomile, Earl Grey, ginger, green, honey bush, lemon balm, lemon verbena, lemongrass, mint, orange spice, rose, white
Condiments	Barbecue sauce, chutney, ketchup, mustard, soy sauce, vinegar (balsamic, apple cider, red wine, white wine)
Seasonings	Allspice, basil, black pepper, cardamom, cayenne, cinnamon, cloves, coriander, curry, fennel, ginger, marjoram, mint, oregano, rosemary, saffron, sage, summer savory, thyme

Herbs of Provence, American Style

Once upon a time, an authentic blend of herbes de Provence included only four—possibly five—native Provençal herbs. But opinions vary wildly on what those herbs were. Some sources declare rosemary, summer savory, oregano, and thyme to be the only pedigreed blend, certified Label Rouge. The one thing agreed on is that lavender was *not* an ingredient of the original Provençal blend—but has since become an essential part of any American mixture of herbs from Provence.

Today the ambiguous seasoning can hold half a dozen—or even a dozen—aromatic herbs associated with the South of France. If you feel adventurous and the taste suits the dish you are preparing, feel free to add an extra Provençal herb or two: basil, marjoram, sage, fennel, parsley, oregano, bay leaf, tarragon, chervil, or mint.

4 teaspoons dried rosemary

4 teaspoons ground dried summer savory (also labeled as ground savory)

4 teaspoons dried oregano

1 tablespoon dried thyme

2 teaspoons dried culinary *L. angustifolia* lavender buds

MAKES ABOUT ⅓ CUP

+ Using a spice grinder or mortar and pestle, coarsely grind the herbs.

+ In a small bowl, mix the herbs together. Pour into an airtight jar or other container.

+ Seal and store in a cool, dark place.

+ Suggestions for use: Consider mixing 1 to 2 tablespoons with olive oil to coat root vegetables or chicken before roasting or grilling. And if you make French ratatouille, herbs of Provence are a must.

Lavender-Peppercorn Medley

Pepper and lavender are quite the power couple in a kitchen. The floral punch of lavender is equal to the bite of pepper, and their yin-yang adds a robust accent to such foods as fresh tomato or cucumber slices, roasted or fried potatoes, grilled fish, scrambled eggs, and green salads. And how about a big bowl of lavender-pepper popcorn!

If fitting to your dish, consider adding a few more layers of flavor into the mix: dried minced onion, mustard seeds, allspice berries, coriander seeds, fennel seeds, and garlic flakes all play well with pepper grinders and lavender.

¾ cup peppercorns (four-peppercorn blend, rainbow, or a combination of Tellicherry, white, and green)
1 tablespoon dried culinary 'Provence' lavandin buds

MAKES ¾ CUP

◆ Combine the peppercorns and lavandin in a small mixing bowl and stir to incorporate.

◆ Pour the mixture into a pepper grinder and use for seasoning as desired.

Lavender Sea Salt

Lavender salt makes a tasty rim on cocktail glasses, a topping for fresh melons, or a savory rub for meats and roasted vegetables. And a jar of this flavorful infused salt makes a lovely handmade gift!

1 cup pink Himalayan salt or other favorite coarse-grain salt

1 tablespoon dried lemon zest (optional)

1 to 2 teaspoons dried culinary *L. angustifolia* lavender buds

MAKES 1 CUP

• Put the salt in a small mixing bowl and set aside.

• In a spice grinder or single-serve food processor, combine the lemon zest and 1 teaspoon of the lavender. Grind for 5 to 10 seconds.

• Transfer the lemon-lavender mixture to the bowl of salt and whisk well to incorporate. Taste-test and add more lavender if desired. Whisk again to blend the flavors.

• Pour the mixture into a salt grinder, or store in a container with an airtight lid. Use for seasoning as desired.

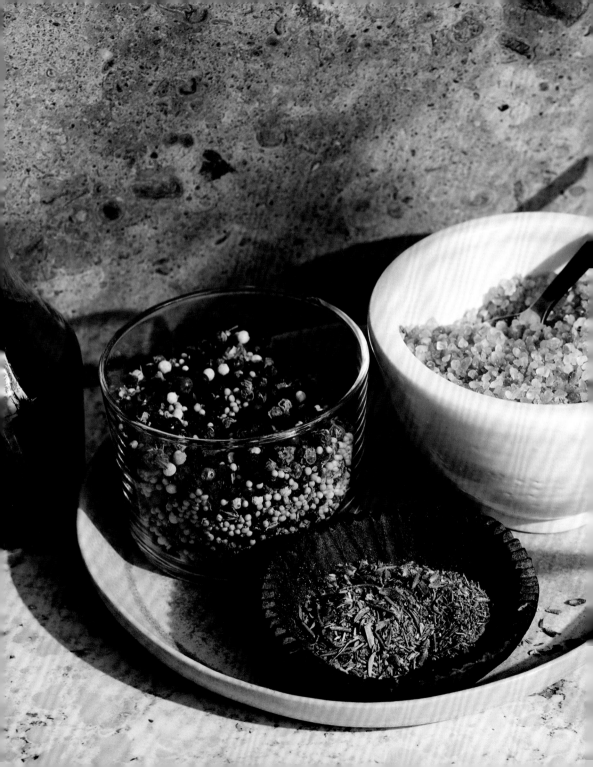

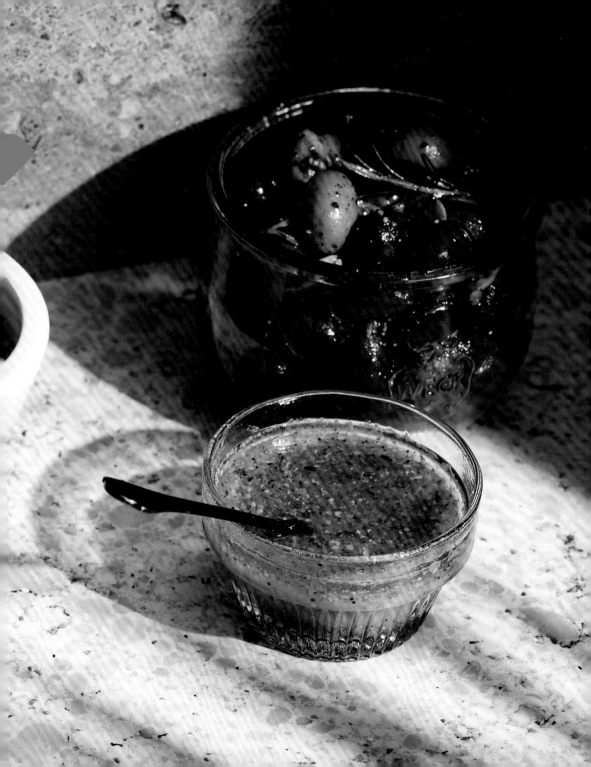

Poppy Seed & Lavender Vinaigrette

This is the perfect topping for a bowl of garden-fresh flavors and colors. Toss it into a mixed salad with spring greens, avocados, strawberries, and coconut. Or dress up a melon, blueberry, and kiwi fruit salad. Or coat a broccoli, olive, and red-onion pasta salad. And for a hearty one-dish meal, crumble in a little feta cheese or add some chickpeas or leftover chicken.

¼ cup light-tasting extra-virgin olive oil

¼ cup white wine or champagne vinegar

2 tablespoons honey

2 teaspoons stone-ground mustard

2 garlic cloves, minced

½ teaspoon poppy seeds

½ teaspoon dried and finely ground culinary *L. angustifolia* lavender buds

MAKES ABOUT 6 SERVINGS

• In a 6- or 8-ounce bottle, combine all the ingredients together. Secure the lid and shake well.

• Serve in a shaker bottle or in a bowl with a spoon. Remix before dressing your salad.

Lavender-Marinated Olives

To make this savory Mediterranean treat for snacking and sharing, toss in your favorite black, green, or purple olives. For best results, choose whole, unpitted olives when available, and then smash and pit them yourself. That way the olives will soak up your marinade instead of the briny solution they were packed in. Feel free to substitute pitted olives if whole olives are not available.

MAKES 3 CUPS

3 cups whole, unpitted olives, such as black, green Castelvetrano, Manzanilla, Kalamata, Niçoise, or Picholine

2 tablespoons freshly squeezed lemon juice (from 1 medium lemon)

1 tablespoon red wine vinegar

1 teaspoon dried culinary *L. angustifolia* lavender buds

½ teaspoon freshly ground Tellicherry pepper

⅓ cup extra-virgin olive oil

2 cloves garlic, slivered or thinly sliced

3 sprigs fresh thyme

3 sprigs fresh rosemary, bruised

• To remove the pits, place the olives on a cutting board. Use the flat side of a large knife to firmly press down on each olive just until it splits and the pit can be easily pulled out.

• In a medium bowl or 1-quart jar, combine the olives, lemon juice, and vinegar. Set aside.

• Using a spice grinder, coarsely grind the lavender and pepper.

• In a small saucepan over the lowest heat, warm the oil. Add the lavender blend, garlic, and sprigs of thyme and rosemary. Cook for 10 minutes.

• Pour the oil mixture over the olives. Stir gently to combine.

• Cool to room temperature, cover, and refrigerate for 1 week before serving.

• To serve, bring to room temperature. Stir gently and remove herb stems. Drain off excess marinade. Serve with chunks of feta cheese if desired.

Lavender-Turmeric Mustard

Mustard seeds, turmeric roots, and lavender flowers all contain anti-inflammatory and antioxidant properties, and they blend well to make a heart-healthy, full-flavored seasoning. You can tailor the heat of your homemade mustard by substituting lighter or darker seeds. A bowl of scorching curry is typically made with black seeds. Artisan mustards tend to favor brown seeds, and mustard in a yellow squeeze bottle is made with mild yellow seeds. You can also choose the texture of the mustard during the grinding process.

4½ tablespoons yellow mustard seeds, divided

1 tablespoon brown mustard seeds (or use yellow mustard seeds for less heat)

1 teaspoon dried culinary *L. angustifolia* lavender buds

½ teaspoon kosher salt

½ teaspoon dried ground turmeric

¼ cup white wine or white grape juice, plus more as needed

¼ cup white wine vinegar, plus more as needed

MAKES 1 CUP

◆ For mustard with a whole-grain texture: In a spice mill, first combine 2 tablespoons of the yellow mustard seeds, the brown seeds, lavender, and salt. Coarsely grind, enough to crack the seeds. Transfer the blend to an 8-ounce jar or bowl. Then grind the remaining 2½ tablespoons of the yellow seeds to a powder. Add to the jar and mix with the cracked blend until incorporated.

◆ For mustard with a smooth texture: In a spice mill, grind all the yellow and brown mustard seeds, lavender, and salt to a powder. Transfer the mixture to an 8-ounce jar or bowl.

◆ Add the turmeric and wine to the jar of grainy or smooth seeds. Stir to blend. Note that cold liquid will spark the heat of crushed seeds, whereas hot liquid will dispel some of their heat.

◆ Cover the jar and let the seasonings steep for 15 minutes at room temperature. Test for spicy heat. Steep longer (up to a day) until the desired level of mildness is reached. The longer the soak, the milder the final flavor.

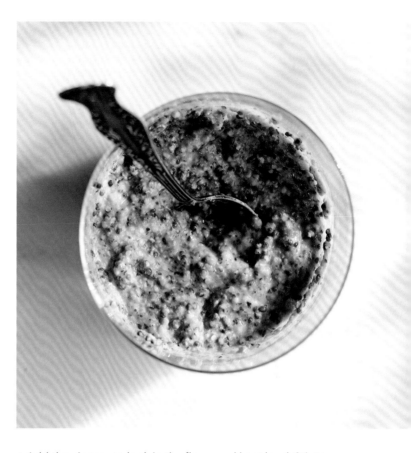

✦ Add the vinegar to lock in the flavor and heat level. Stir to mix. If you ground all the seeds to a powder, you may need to add a bit more wine and vinegar in equal amounts to thin the consistency.

✦ Cover and refrigerate for at least a full day. A week is even better. Don't skip this step! Mustard is sharply bitter when the flavors are first introduced but mellows as the flavors marry.

Lavender-Infused Oils & Vinegars

The scent and flavor of lavender flowers come from lavender's essential oil. Some of that fragrant oil can be coaxed from flowers in a medium of vinegar or warm oil. For a base oil of DIY skin-care products, infuse lavender into your choice of carrier oil (see Popular Essential Oil Carriers on page 60). For use in culinary recipes, choose an unrefined oil, such as olive, avocado, or sunflower. For lavender-infused vinegar, go with apple cider, white wine, or champagne vinegar for best flavor results.

Whichever medium you infuse with lavender, always use a dry, sterile jar and lid. Be sure lavender buds are completely dry too, because moisture within flowers could cause mold or bacteria to grow in your infusion.

MAKES 1 CUP

1 cup plant-based culinary oil, carrier oil, or vinegar of your choice
½ cup dried culinary *L. angustifolia* lavender or lavandin buds

FOR INFUSED OIL

• In a small glass or ceramic frying pan or saucepan over medium heat, add the oil. (Alternatively, warm the oil in a heatproof glass measuring cup or canning jar placed inside a metal pan with 1 inch of water.) Bring the temperature of the oil to about 175 degrees F. If bubbles begin to form in the oil, the temperature is too hot.

- In the pan or a separate bowl, using the back of a spoon, bruise the lavender buds to release more of their scent. Add the lavender to the oil. Bloom the lavender buds in the hot oil until fragrant, 30 to 60 minutes. Olive oil and other oils with a strong scent of their own may need to infuse longer than oils with a neutral scent.

- Remove from heat and allow to cool. With a fine-mesh sieve, strain out the buds as you pour the oil into an 8-ounce jar.

- Store the infused oil in the refrigerator. For skin-care products used at room temperature, you can slow oxidation and extend shelf life by adding a few drops of vitamin E oil.

FOR INFUSED VINEGAR

- Into an 8-ounce jar, add the lavender buds and pour the vinegar over them.

- Place in a dark cupboard for 2 to 12 weeks, depending on the strength of the lavender infusion you want.

- Check each week. Strain out the buds when the fragrance of the vinegar appeals to you.

Lavender Sugar

A light sprinkling of this floral sugar complements a bowl of fresh berries or peaches, replaces syrup over a plate of your favorite French toast, and gives ordinary oatmeal cookies a dash of extraordinary flavor. And try adding a teaspoon of lavender sweetness to a mug of mint, ginger, or orange-spice tea!

1 cup sugar
½ to 1 teaspoon dried culinary *L. angustifolia* lavender buds

MAKES 1¼ CUPS

◆ Into a clean, small spice or coffee grinder, pour the sugar and ½ teaspoon of the lavender buds.

◆ Process for 1 minute, until the sugar crystals resemble a fine flour. The consistency will be of superfine sugar (castor sugar in the UK; *sucre en poudre* in France), which dissolves easily and melts in your mouth the way powdered sugar does, but without any cornstarch.

◆ Taste-test and add more lavender if desired. Process again until incorporated.

◆ Store in a tightly covered container away from humidity.

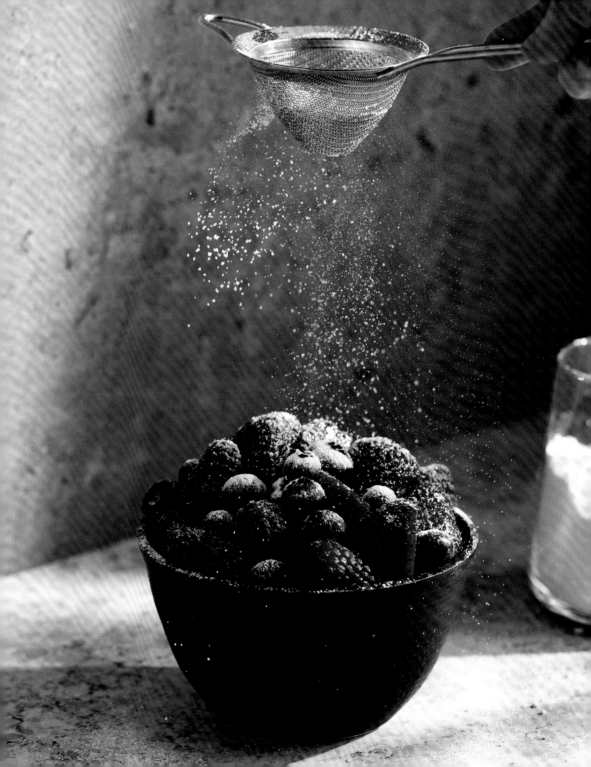

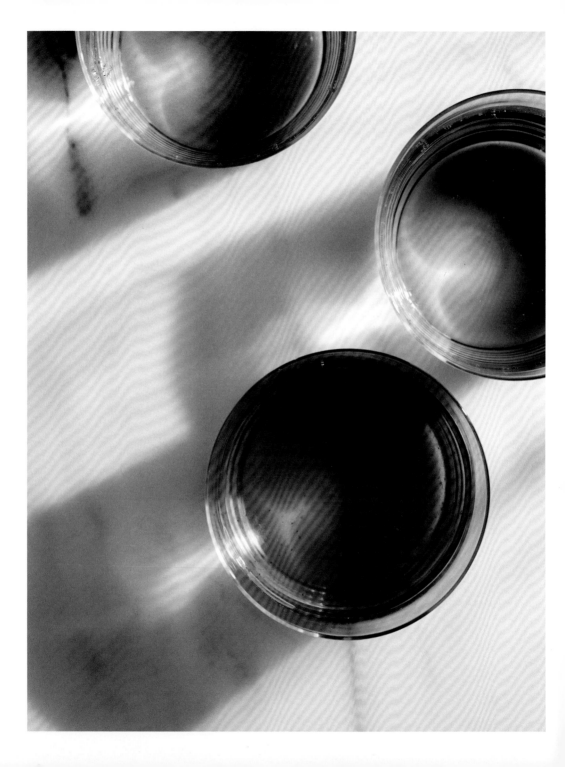

Lavender Simple Syrup

When cocktails or dessert glazes call for simple syrup, an infusion of lavender can add a subtle floral note. The color of the syrup may vary, ranging from hazy purple to herbal-tea brown to a healthy shade of green.

¼ cup dried culinary *L. angustifolia* lavender buds

1 cup water

1 cup granulated sugar, demerara sugar (for a light toffee flavor), turbinado sugar (for a mild caramel flavor), honey, or other sweetener

The color of lavender syrup is affected by the quantity of buds, variety of lavender, and type of pan you use. Be sure to avoid reactive pans, such as aluminum, cast iron, and copper. If you're hoping for syrup with a purple hue, choose dark-purple buds, such as 'Royal Velvet'. But no matter the color, your kitchen will smell amazing!

MAKES 1½ CUPS

◆ Put the lavender buds in a small glass or stainless-steel saucepan. Bruise the buds with the back of a spoon.

◆ Add the water and sugar. Over high heat, bring the mixture almost to a boil. Remove from heat and stir until the sweetener dissolves.

◆ Cover and let steep for 30 to 60 minutes, until the desired lavender fragrance and taste is reached. Flavor will strengthen while steeping.

◆ Through a fine-mesh sieve, pour the syrup into a sterilized 12-ounce jar.

◆ Cap tightly and store in the refrigerator. The syrup should keep for about a month. You can double its storage life by adding 1 ounce of vodka to the syrup, if desired.

◆ To use the syrup in beverages, substitute about 1½ teaspoons of lavender syrup for 1 teaspoon of sugar. To cut the tartness of fruit, drizzle the syrup over poached or fresh fruit. As a sweet foil to a savory marinade or dressing, add a little lavender syrup. To moisten and flavor cakes, use a fork to perforate the top of each layer and drip lavender syrup into the holes.

Lavender-Infused Milks & Creams

Infusing the summery scent of lavender into milks or creams is as simple as brewing tea. By first steeping and then straining out the lavender pieces, you can impart the flavor and scent of lavender into plant-based or dairy beverages without any bitter aftertaste from the buds.

For a batch of fresh, natural lavender whipped cream, add a tablespoon of powdered sugar to a cup of chilled lavender-infused cream (dairy or coconut). Beat in a chilled bowl until stiff peaks form. For a refreshing dessert, mix lavender whipped cream 1:1 with yogurt, and then layer the creamy mixture with berries.

1 cup milk, nondairy milk, or cream (for whipping, use heavy dairy cream or coconut cream)
1½ teaspoons dried culinary *L. angustifolia* lavender buds

MAKES 1 CUP

◆ In a small saucepan, bring the milk just to a simmer and remove from heat immediately.

◆ Add the lavender buds, cover the pan, and let steep for 30 to 60 minutes, until the desired level of lavender fragrance and flavor is reached.

◆ Using a fine-mesh sieve, strain out the buds. Refrigerate the milk overnight, or for at least 6 hours.

◆ Use the steeped milk in coffee, tea, or hot chocolate.

Lavender & Honey Coconut Butter

This garden-inspired butter is delicious when slathered on a piece of warm cornbread fresh from the oven. For an eye-catching presentation, sprinkle fresh lavender petals over the peaks of your creamy whipped butter.

5 tablespoons virgin (unrefined) coconut oil

3 tablespoons canola or sunflower oil

¼ teaspoon fine kosher salt

¼ cup honey or pure maple syrup

1 teaspoon dried and finely ground culinary *L. angustifolia* lavender buds

Zest of 1 medium navel orange (optional)

MAKES ½ CUP

◆ In a medium bowl, blend together the oils and salt. Chill in the refrigerator for 20 to 30 minutes.

◆ Add the honey, lavender, and orange zest.

◆ With an electric mixer or hand whisk, whip together all the ingredients until light and fluffy.

◆ Transfer the coconut butter to a small serving dish and serve soft. Cover and store any unused butter in the refrigerator for up to 2 weeks.

Lavender-Fig Jam

Like apples and cinnamon or peaches and cream, the pairing of figs and lavender creates a harmony that lures the senses. If you're not a fan of figs, this jam is equally tasty made with dried berries.

For a sweet and savory grilled sandwich, butter up some cinnamon-raisin bread, spread with goat cheese and a bit of this lavender-fig jam, and grill over medium heat until golden.

½ cup water
4 ounces dried Smyrna, California golden, or Calimyrna figs, stemmed (not Mission figs)
½ teaspoon dried and finely ground culinary *L. angustifolia* lavender buds
½ teaspoon lemon zest
¼ cup sugar
1 tablespoon freshly squeezed lemon juice
Pinch of salt

MAKES ⅔ CUP

◆ In a small saucepan over medium-high heat, add the water, dried figs, lavender, and lemon zest. Bring to a boil.

◆ Remove from heat, cover, and let stand for 30 minutes to soften and plump up the figs.

◆ With a slotted spoon, transfer the figs to a cutting board. Reserve the liquid in the pan.

◆ Using a sharp knife, chop the figs into small pieces. The larger the pieces, the chunkier the jam will be. If you prefer a smoother jam, mince the figs.

◆ Add the sugar and lemon juice to the saucepan. Bring to a boil and stir to dissolve the sugar.

◆ Add the chopped figs and salt. Bring to a boil again, and then reduce heat and simmer until thickened, 15 to 20 minutes.

◆ Remove from heat and allow to cool. Transfer to a serving bowl or clean jar.

◆ Jam should keep in the refrigerator for a few weeks.

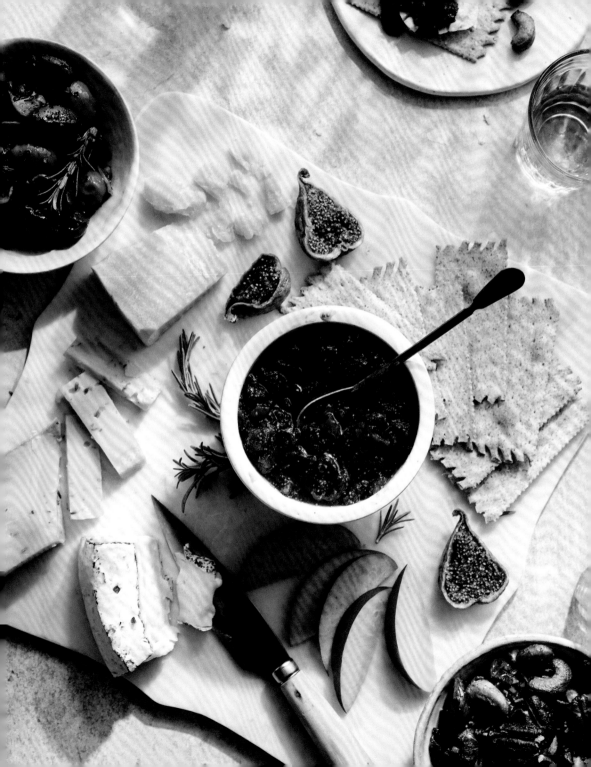

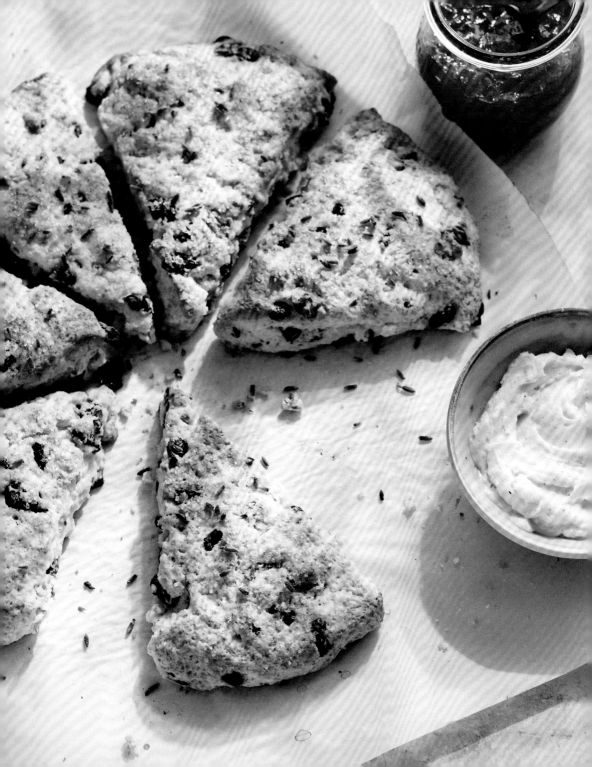

Apricot-Lavender Scones

The scent of baking apricots and lavender will add a kind of aromatherapy to your morning! These butter-free goodies have half the saturated fat as typical scones, with every bit as much flavor. Frozen wedges of scone dough offer easy morning baking too. Simply defrost the wedges for about an hour and pop them into the oven.

Powdered sugar, sifted, for dusting
2 cups all-purpose flour
⅓ cup sugar
1 tablespoon baking powder
¼ teaspoon fine kosher salt (optional)
½ cup (about 3 ounces) chopped dried apricots
½ cup dried cranberries
½ cup (about 2 ounces) chopped walnuts
1⅓ cups Lavender-Infused Cream (page 150), plus more as needed
¼ teaspoon dried purple culinary *L. angustifolia* lavender buds
Demerara sugar, for sprinkling
Lavender & Honey Coconut Butter (page 151), lavender-infused whipped cream (page 150), or jam, for serving (optional)

MAKES 8 SCONES

◆ Preheat the oven to 400 degrees F. Line a large baking sheet with parchment paper. Dust a work surface or nonstick pastry mat with powdered sugar.

◆ In a large bowl, combine the flour, sugar, baking powder, and salt and mix well with a sturdy spoon.

◆ Stir in the apricots, cranberries, and walnuts. Break up any clumps while incorporating into the dry ingredients. Add the cream and stir just until blended.

◆ Place the dough onto the dusted work surface and knead until smooth—about a dozen cycles of pressing, folding, and turning. If needed to create a cohesive dough, add more cream, 1 tablespoon at a time.

◆ Press and shape the dough into a circle about 1 inch thick. Sprinkle the lavender buds and demerara sugar over the top. With a sharp knife, cut the circle into 8 wedges. Transfer the wedges to the baking sheet. (To bake later, transfer them into a freezer storage bag.)

◆ Bake for about 18 minutes, until golden brown. A toothpick inserted into the center should come out clean.

◆ Serve warm with butter, whipped cream, or jam, if desired.

Baked Pear & Lavender Pancakes

If you were to cross a German pancake with a French baked custard, the result might be this deliciously puffy and fruity pancake. For even more dazzle, add some bright pansies, rose petals, or fresh berries to your garnish.

1 cup water

⅓ cup sugar

1 teaspoon dried purple culinary *L. angustifolia* lavender buds

3 large or 4 medium fresh Anjou or Bosc pears

¼ cup unsalted butter, melted and divided

4 eggs

½ cup all-purpose flour

½ cup light brown or dark brown sugar

2 teaspoons vanilla extract

⅛ teaspoon lemon extract

⅛ teaspoon fine kosher salt (optional)

¾ cup light pear syrup, reserved from pan

1 medium lemon, cut into 6 wedges

Powdered sugar, sifted, for dusting

MAKES 6 SERVINGS

✦ In a medium saucepan, combine the water, sugar, and lavender. Stir to dissolve the sugar. With a sharp knife, core and slice pears about ¼ inch thick. Add the pear slices to the pan.

✦ Over medium-high heat, bring the mixture to a boil and cook for 2 minutes. Remove from heat and cover. Steep for 10 minutes to infuse lavender flavor into the pear syrup.

✦ Holding a small fine-mesh sieve over a measuring cup, strain ¾ cup of the syrup into the cup. Set aside.

✦ While the syrup cools, preheat the oven to 350 degrees F.

✦ Prepare 6 (10-ounce) individual baking dishes or a 9-inch pie pan by spraying the edges with nonstick spray and then coating the bottom of each dish with ½ teaspoon of melted butter. Arrange the pear slices to cover the bottoms of the dishes.

✦ In a blender, whip the eggs on medium speed until frothy, about 30 seconds. Add the flour, brown sugar, vanilla, lemon extract, and salt. Blend until the batter is smooth and thick, about 2 minutes. Stop to scrape the sides as needed.

✦ Add the pear syrup and the remaining 3 tablespoons of butter to the batter. Blend until smooth, about 15 seconds.

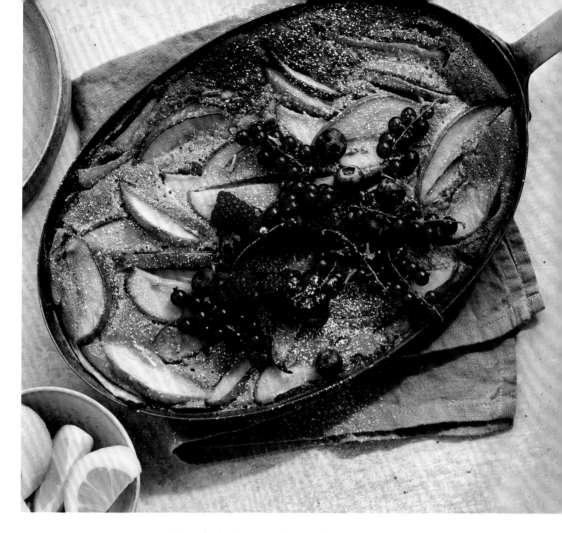

◆ Pour the batter evenly over the pears and bake uncovered for 20 to 25 minutes, until golden brown and fluffy. For the 9-inch pie pan, increase the cooking time to about 30 minutes.

◆ To serve, top each dish with a squeeze of lemon juice and a sprinkle of powdered sugar. Garnish with a sprig of lavender and a few berries or edible flowers if desired. Serve immediately.

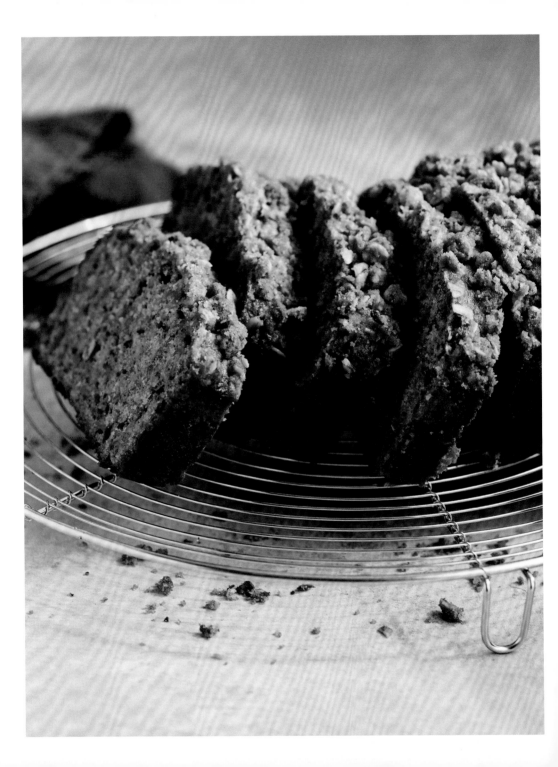

Chai Spice & Lavender Zucchini Bread

Chai spices fuse with lavender and lemon for a fresh burst of flavor in this naturally moist summer favorite. If you don't have chai spice on hand, take a minute to make the Chai Spice Blend on page 160 before you start on the bread. You'll have enough spice blend for 2 loaves, so you can also double the batter and freeze a loaf for later.

For the bread

⅔ cup whole wheat flour

⅔ cup all-purpose flour

1 teaspoon baking powder

1 teaspoon Chai Spice Blend (recipe follows)

½ teaspoon baking soda

¼ teaspoon fine kosher salt

⅓ cup old-fashioned oats

1 teaspoon dried and finely ground culinary *L. angustifolia* lavender buds

2 eggs

½ cup raw sugar

½ cup avocado oil

¼ cup pure maple syrup

1½ teaspoons pure vanilla extract

Juice (2 tablespoons) and zest from 1 medium lemon

1 cup unpeeled, grated fresh zucchini, firmly packed (squeeze out excess liquid)

MAKES 1 LOAF

• Preheat the oven to 350 degrees F. Coat a 1½-quart loaf pan with coconut oil or nonstick spray.

• In a medium bowl, sift together the flours, baking powder, spices, baking soda, and salt. Add the oats and lavender, mix well, and set aside.

• In a large bowl, mix the eggs, sugar, avocado oil, maple syrup, vanilla, lemon juice, and zest. Stir in the zucchini.

• Fold in the dry ingredients, stirring just until combined. Do not overmix.

• Pour the batter into the pan, and bake for 40 minutes.

⟶

For the topping

2 tablespoons virgin (unrefined) coconut oil, melted

2 tablespoons old-fashioned oats

2 tablespoons packed light brown sugar or sweetener of choice

1 to 2 tablespoons all-purpose flour

½ teaspoon dried culinary *L. angustifolia* lavender buds (optional)

¼ teaspoon Chai Spice Blend (recipe follows)

◆ While the bread is baking, make the topping. In a small bowl, whisk the coconut oil, oats, brown sugar, flour, lavender, and chai spice. (For a more traditional streusel texture, grind the oats in a blender first and then mix with the remaining ingredients.)

◆ Remove the bread from the oven, sprinkle with the topping, and return the pan to the oven. Bake for 10 to 15 minutes more, or until a toothpick inserted in the middle comes out clean.

◆ Cool on a wire rack. Serve warm. To freeze, cool completely and remove from the pan. Cover with plastic wrap and then seal in foil or a freezer bag.

Chai Spice Blend

4 teaspoons ground cinnamon

3 teaspoons ground ginger

1½ teaspoons ground cardamom

¼ teaspoon ground cloves

¼ teaspoon ground nutmeg

¼ teaspoon ground black pepper

After baking the bread, use any leftover homemade chai spice to make lavender-chai lattes! In a mug, mix ½ teaspoon of the blend with ½ teaspoon dried and finely ground culinary lavender buds in ¼ cup hot water. Sweeten to taste. Top off with steamed coconut milk.

MAKES 3 TABLESPOONS

◆ In a small bowl, combine all the spices and mix well.

◆ Store any unused chai spice in an airtight jar.

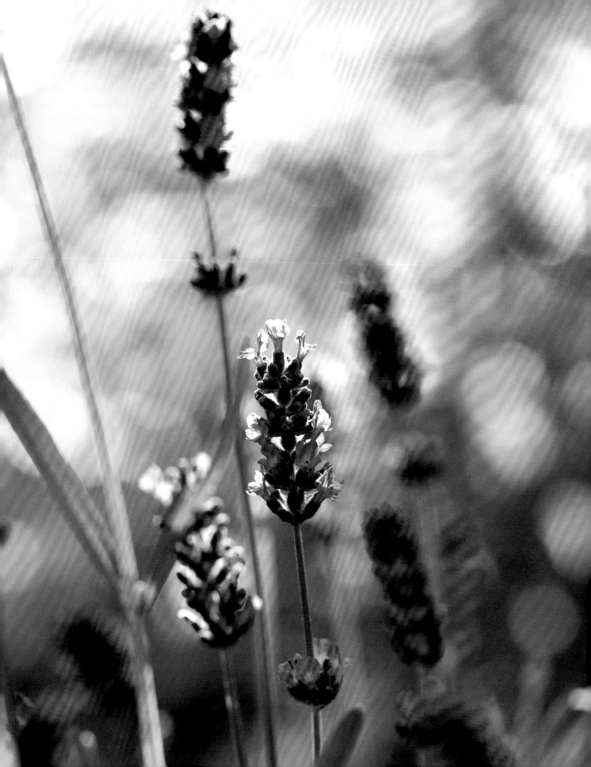

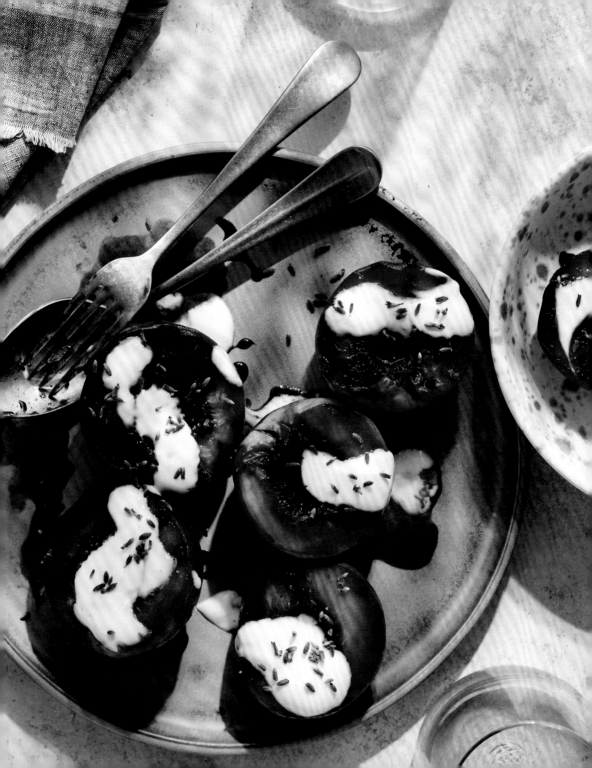

Lavender-Balsamic Grilled Peaches

This lavender glaze drizzled over peaches is a deeply flavored balsamic reduction that can also baste fresh salmon fillets, marinate chicken breasts, and smartly dress a spinach salad. Double the recipe, and the extra glaze will keep in the refrigerator for several weeks.

MAKES 2 SERVINGS

For the glaze
1 cup Modena balsamic vinegar
⅓ cup honey
1½ teaspoons dried culinary *L. angustifolia* lavender buds

For the peaches
2 ripe but firm freestone peaches or nectarines, cut in half and pitted
1 tablespoon light brown sugar, divided
1 tablespoon honey
¼ cup plain Greek yogurt

• To make the glaze, in a small saucepan over medium heat, combine the vinegar, honey, and lavender. Stir often. When bubbling begins, reduce heat and simmer until reduced by half, 10 to 15 minutes. Remove from heat, cover, and allow the mixture to cool, thicken, and absorb the flavor of lavender. Strain before using.

• To prepare the peaches, in a grilling pan over medium-high heat, or on an outdoor grill, place the peach halves cut side up and sprinkle them with half the brown sugar. Turn them over and cook for 2 to 3 minutes, until they release a little juice and show blackened grill marks.

• Sprinkle the other side of the peaches with the remaining brown sugar. Turn them over and cook for another 2 to 3 minutes.

• Place the peach halves, cut side up, onto 2 small plates. Drizzle the lavender-balsamic glaze over the peaches.

• In a small bowl, stir the honey into the yogurt, and top each peach with a dollop of sweetened yogurt.

• Garnish with lavender blossoms or dark-purple culinary lavender buds, and serve warm.

Maple-Glazed Nuts with Lavender & Cayenne

Bake up a heart-healthy batch of crunchy nuts wrapped in maple and lavender deliciousness. This vegan-friendly, protein-rich snack is a sweet and spicy treat for lunchboxes, and for adding some zing to your trail mix.

6 tablespoons pure maple syrup
2 teaspoons dried culinary *L. angustifolia* lavender buds
½ teaspoon cayenne pepper
½ teaspoon kosher salt (optional)
2 cups unsalted or salted cashews, pecans, or mixed nuts

MAKES 2 CUPS

◆ Position a rack in the center of the oven and preheat to 350 degrees F. Line a large baking sheet with parchment paper.

◆ In a small bowl, whisk together the maple syrup, lavender, cayenne, and salt. Add the nuts and stir gently to coat evenly.

◆ Transfer the coated nuts to the prepared baking sheet. With a rubber spatula, spread the nuts in a single layer and then scrape any remaining glaze from the bowl over the nuts.

◆ Bake for 10 to 12 minutes. The glaze should be browned but not burnt. If the tops of the nuts are sticky to the touch, return the pan to the oven and check for doneness again after 1 minute.

◆ Remove from the oven and carefully slide the parchment with the nuts onto a wire rack. Let cool.

◆ Once the caramelized coating has cooled and hardened, break apart the nut clusters and store in an airtight container.

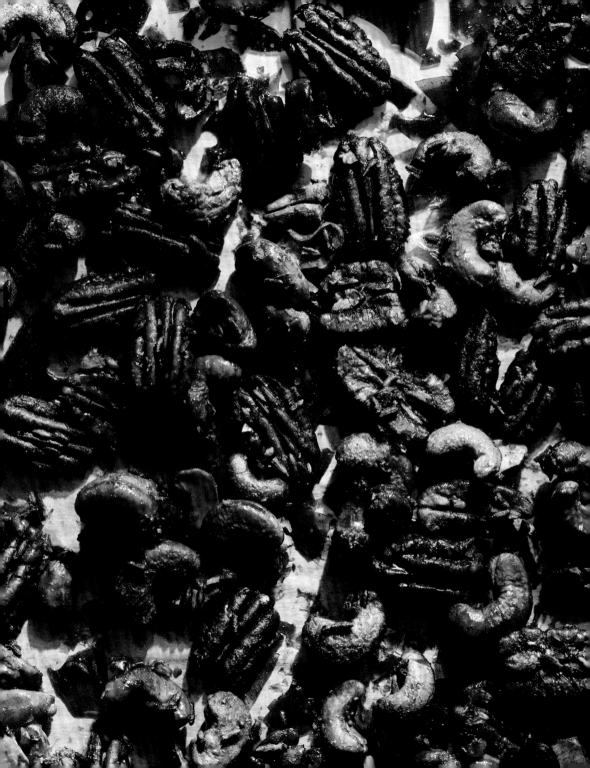

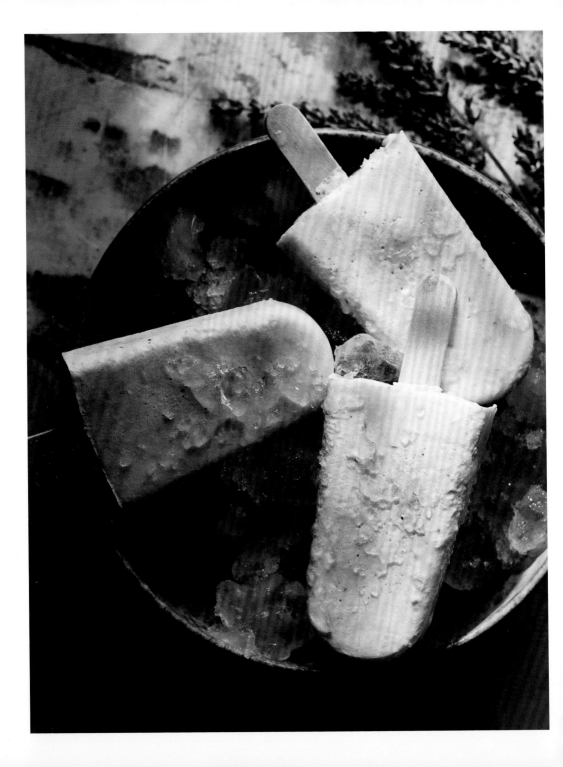

Lime-Lavender Coconut Pops

Tart, refreshing, and natural, these frozen pops can brighten any sultry summer afternoon. If you don't have molds for ice pops, you can pour the mixture into paper cups or a large silicone ice cube tray. Natural craft sticks or small wooden spoons make great Popsicle sticks.

1 (13.5-ounce) can full-fat unsweetened coconut milk (do not use low-fat milk from a carton)

Juice and some pulp of 1 medium lime

2½ tablespoons pure maple syrup

1 teaspoon dried or 1½ teaspoons fresh culinary *L. angustifolia* lavender buds

MAKES 6 (3-OUNCE) POPS

◆ In a blender, combine all the ingredients. Blend at high speed for 1 minute.

◆ Pour into 6 ice pop molds. Place in the freezer for about 1 hour, until the pops are hardened enough to hold the sticks in place. Insert the sticks and freeze until fully hardened.

◆ For best results, eat immediately. If frozen too long, coconut milk will separate into layers. Depending on your molds, you may need to dip the bases under warm water until they release the pops.

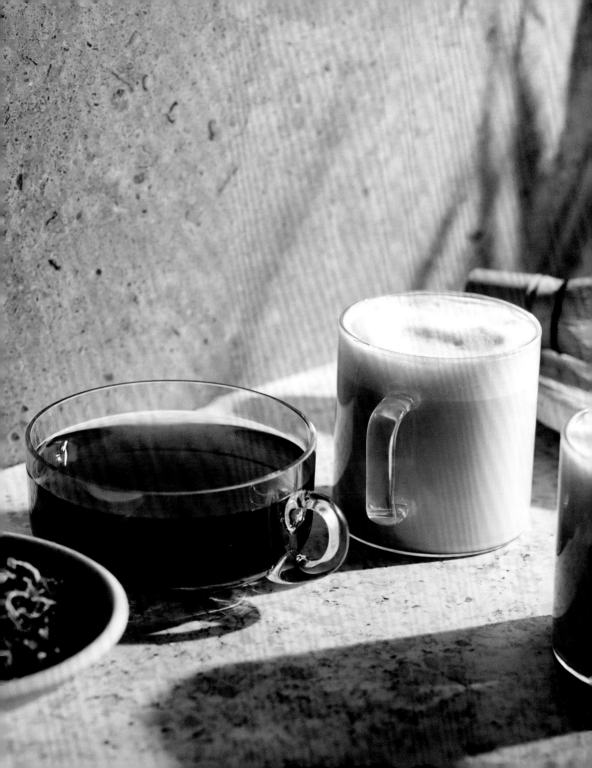

Fresh-Start Tea with Earl Grey, Lavender & Citrus

Teas made from garden-gathered ingredients let your body gently and naturally absorb some of the healing compounds of lavender and other aromatic plants.[1] This blend of Earl Grey and lavender with a bright touch of citrus can jump-start a mindset of calm acuity. To dry your own antioxidant-rich citrus zest for this blend, see page 170.

½ cup Dried Citrus Zest (recipe follows)
½ cup dried culinary *L. angustifolia* lavender buds
¼ cup loose, dried Earl Grey tea leaves
Sweetener of your choice (optional)

MAKES 8 OUNCES LOOSE-LEAF TEA (ENOUGH FOR 16 SERVINGS)

• Combine the citrus zest, lavender buds, and tea in a bowl. Stir gently to blend.

• Transfer to an 8-ounce jar or an airtight container and tightly close the lid.

• To prepare a cup of tea, add 1 tablespoon of the tea blend to a tea strainer, ball, or drawstring muslin bag. Pour 10 ounces (1¼ cups) of boiling water into a cup, and lower the strainer into the hot water. Cover to retain the volatile, nourishing components of the oils, and steep for 5 to 10 minutes. Add sweetener to taste if desired. (Don't add milk, as citrus can cause milk to curdle.)

Dried Citrus Zest

Citrus rinds are full of immune-supporting vitamin C, plus D-limonene and its antioxidant properties. Whenever fresh orange, lemon, or lime juice is part of your menu, you can dry the zest for later use.

2 medium organic lemons
2 medium organic limes
1 medium organic navel
   orange

MAKES ABOUT ½ CUP

• Scrub away any wax coating on the fruit.

• Zest each rind using a citrus zester or microplane grater to remove a shallow layer of peel: Over a small bowl, hold the zester firmly against the skin of the fruit, and drag the zester from the top to the bottom of the fruit. Leave behind the bitter white pith under the rind.

• To dry in a food dehydrator, transfer the zest to the fruit-leather tray, or arrange on a tray lined with parchment paper. The ideal temperature for drying fine citrus zest is the lowest setting, about 95 degrees F. Dry for 4 to 6 hours, until crisp. If you don't have a food dehydrator, spread the grated peels on a baking sheet lined with parchment paper and allow to air-dry away from direct sunlight for about 2 days. (Oven- and microwave-drying tend to cause uneven scorching with citrus zest and are not recommended.)

• Cool completely and store the fully dried zest in an airtight container in a cool, dark place for up to a year.

Lavender & Matcha Latte

Under a layer of fragrant, velvety foam lies a calming boost of antioxidants. Be sure to select culinary-grade matcha powder with bright-green color and a fresh, grassy scent. Choose your favorite dairy or nondairy milk. For the best nondairy froth, buy a specially formulated barista-style milk.

¼ cup water

1 teaspoon culinary matcha powder

1 teaspoon sweetener of your choice

¾ cup Lavender-Infused Milk (page 150)

¾ cup plain dairy or nondairy milk

MAKES 2 SERVINGS

✦ Heat the water to about 175 degrees F. If the water is hotter, bitterness will increase.

✦ In a small bowl, combine the water with the matcha powder and the sweetener to taste. With a bamboo matcha whisk or other small whisk, blend to remove all lumps.

✦ With a milk frother, steam the milks together. If your frother does not steam the milk, heat the milk in a microwave first, or heat in a pan on the stove top over low heat while frothing. Remove from heat when you see fine steam rising from the milk. For best results, heat nondairy milks to 125 degrees F and dairy milks to 150 degrees F.

✦ The goal is to create a pourable microfoam of tiny bubbles—not a dry foam with big bubbles. A quick bump on the counter will help pop unwanted large bubbles on top of the foam. Swirl the container or pan to blend the foam into the milk below it.

✦ Slowly pour the foamy milk into 2 mugs, and pour half the matcha mixture over the milk in each mug. Serve immediately.

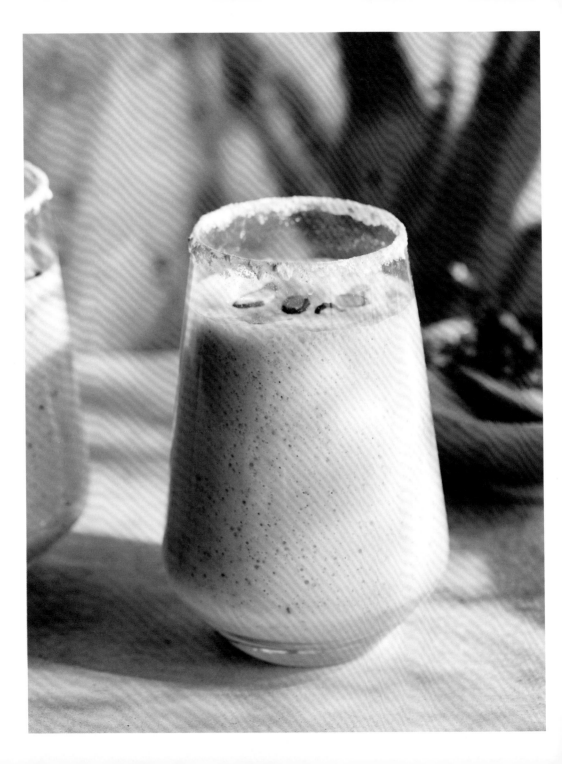

Lavender & Cardamom Lassi

A classic Indian lassi can be sweet or savory, made with or without mango or rose petals, but a lassi is always made with probiotic yogurt and aromatic spices. Some call it the world's oldest smoothie.

Lavender Sugar (page 146; optional)

1 cup plain yogurt or almond milk yogurt

½ cup unsweetened almond or coconut milk

1 ripe nectarine or peach, chilled and sliced, or about 1 cup frozen

2 tablespoons pure maple syrup, plus more as needed

1 teaspoon grated fresh ginger

½ teaspoon ground cardamom

½ to 1 teaspoon dried culinary *L. angustifolia* lavender buds

¼ cup sliced almonds

MAKES 2 SERVINGS

◆ If serving on a warm day, cover and chill the fruit slices in the freezer for a couple of hours or overnight.

◆ Dip the rims of serving glasses in water, then shake off the excess and dip them in lavender sugar.

◆ In a blender, combine the yogurt, milk, fruit, maple syrup, ginger, cardamom, and ½ teaspoon of the lavender. Blend on low speed for about 30 seconds, and then increase to medium-high speed for about 1 minute, or until smooth. Frozen fruit may take longer than fresh. Taste and then mix in additional syrup and lavender if desired. When fully blended, the lassi will be flecked with tiny bits of fruit skin and herbs that hold vital micronutrients and phytochemicals.

◆ To serve, pour the lavender lassi into the prepared glasses. Sprinkle with sliced almonds. Enjoy with breakfast or lunch, after a workout, or as an afternoon treat.

Lavender-Lime Refresher

Every pitcher of this naturally pink drink is a crowd-pleaser. The steeping of deep-purple or dark-blue buds is what lends just enough color to pink-up a batch of this summer essential, and substituting lemon for the lime won't alter the lovely pink color. Serving a cocktail crowd? Double the recipe and stir some honey bourbon, to taste, into your punch bowl.

2 cups water

1¾ cups sugar, or 1 cup agave nectar, or 1¼ cups pure maple syrup

¼ cup fresh culinary dark-purple *L. angustifolia* lavender buds

Fresh grated zest of 1 large lime

1 cup freshly squeezed lime juice (from 8 to 10 large limes)

A few thin slices of lime

MAKES ABOUT 8 (1-CUP) SERVINGS

• In a medium-sized pan over high heat, combine the water, sugar, lavender, and lime zest. Bring to a boil, and then reduce heat to a simmer.

• With a long-handled spoon, stir until the sugar dissolves. Remove from heat and let stand for 10 minutes. Strain out the solids and discard.

• In a 2-liter pitcher, combine the lavender syrup and lime juice. Fill the pitcher with about 6 cups of water and ice to your liking.

• Toss in a few lime slices. Stir and serve.

Lavender Switchel

Switchels, with a cooling, natural vinegar base, were once called "Haymaker's Punch." By the gallon they quenched the thirst of seventeenth-century laborers toiling in hot fields. The delicious hydrating drink can be made either alcoholic or nonalcoholic, and today's variations are served at spas and cocktail parties, and are swigged by gardeners and athletes. This lavender-infused switchel has a kick of ginger, a nip of vinegar, and a kiss of pure maple syrup.

For the switchel

1 tablespoon dried culinary *L. angustifolia* lavender buds
1 cup filtered water
½ cup pure maple syrup
⅓ cup apple cider vinegar
1 (2-inch) piece of ginger, peeled and grated

For serving

3 cups carbonated or still filtered water
1 teaspoon dried and finely ground culinary *L. angustifolia* lavender buds
4 ounces (½ cup) gin or ginger ale

MAKES 4 SERVINGS

◆ To make the switchel, first add the lavender buds to a 1-quart glass or stainless-steel bowl. With the back of a spoon, bruise the lavender to release the oils.

◆ Add the water, maple syrup, vinegar, and grated ginger to the bowl. Stir gently to blend. Cover and refrigerate for at least a day and up to a week.

◆ Strain out the solids and keep the switchel chilled until ready to mix and serve.

◆ To serve, in a 1½-quart pitcher or large jar, mix the switchel, water, and ground lavender. Stir to blend.

◆ Into the serving glasses, add ice, if desired, and 1 ounce of gin or ginger ale. Top off each glass with the blended switchel, and garnish with a sprig of lavender.

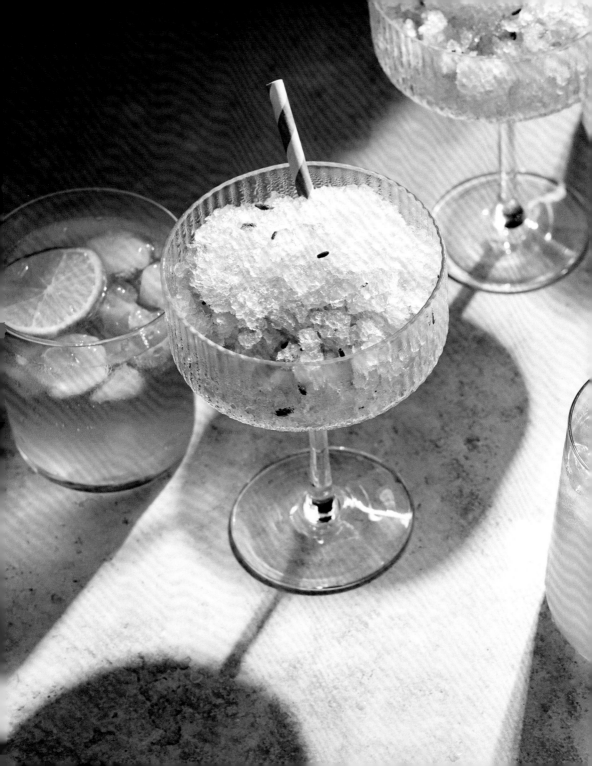

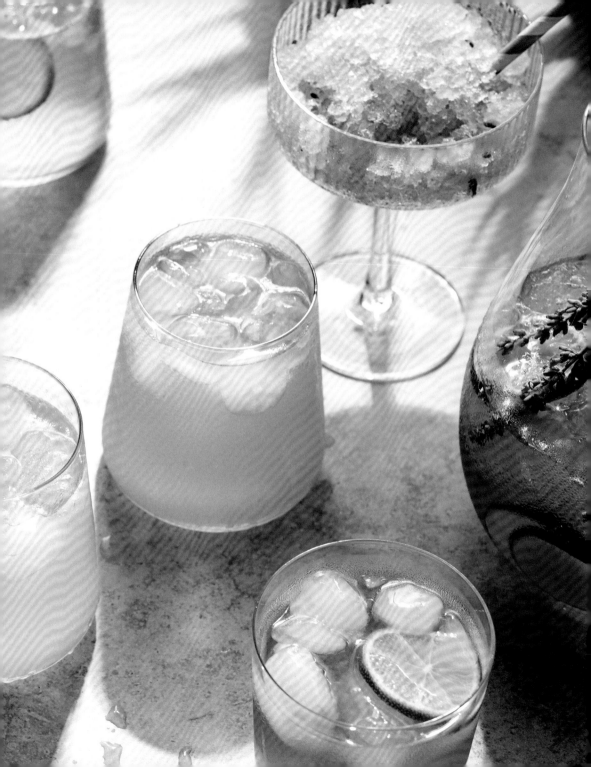

Lavender Frosé

Garden-to-glass cocktails will infuse your relaxation time with icy freshness—especially when the tang of citrus and the bloom of lavender are mixed with the delicate frozen crystals of rosé wine. Go ahead, heap your glass full, garnish with citrus zest, top with a lavender sprig, and relax with a smile at the end of those hot summer days.

2 cups full-bodied
  rosé wine
½ cup Lavender Simple
  Syrup (page 149)
½ cup water or seltzer
  water
¼ cup fresh lemon
  juice (from 2 medium
  lemons)
½ teaspoon dried and
  finely ground culinary
  L. angustifolia lavender
  buds

MAKES 4 SERVINGS

• In a medium mixing bowl, stir together all the ingredients.

• Pour into a 9-by-13-inch pan, cover, and place in the freezer.

• After 30 minutes, use a dinner fork to stir and flake the ice into crystals. Repeat every 30 minutes for about 3 hours, until the mixture is frozen. The recipe can be made several days ahead and frozen covered until ready to serve.

• To serve, remove from the freezer and scoop into wine-glasses. For a slushy, pourable consistency, scoop into a blender and process until smooth before pouring into glasses. Garnish if desired and serve immediately.

Day's-End Tea with Lavender, Ginger & Lemon Balm

Ease out of a busy day with this trio of herbs. Lavender and lemon balm help to quiet the mind and relax tense muscles, while ginger assists with digestion. If you don't enjoy the spicy taste of ginger, an equal portion of dried, crushed peppermint leaves can take its place.

When serving immediately, fresh ginger slices can be substituted for dried slices using a 1:1 ratio. Fresh lemon balm leaves or chamomile flowers can also be used with a 3:1 fresh-to-dry ratio.

2/3 cup Dried Ginger Slices (page 181)

1/3 cup dried culinary *L. angustifolia* lavender buds

1/3 cup dried, crumbled lemon balm (*Melissa officinalis*) or chamomile flowers

Sweetener of your choice (optional)

MAKES 8 OUNCES LOOSE-LEAF TEA (ENOUGH FOR 12 TO 16 SERVINGS)

• Combine the dried herbs in a bowl, stirring gently to blend.

• Transfer to an airtight jar or container.

• To serve, add 1 rounded tablespoon of the dried blend to a tea strainer, ball, or drawstring muslin bag. Pour 10 ounces (1¼ cups) of boiling water into a cup, and lower the strainer into the hot water.

• Cover to retain the volatile, nourishing components of the oils and steep for 5 to 10 minutes.

• Add sweetener to taste if desired.

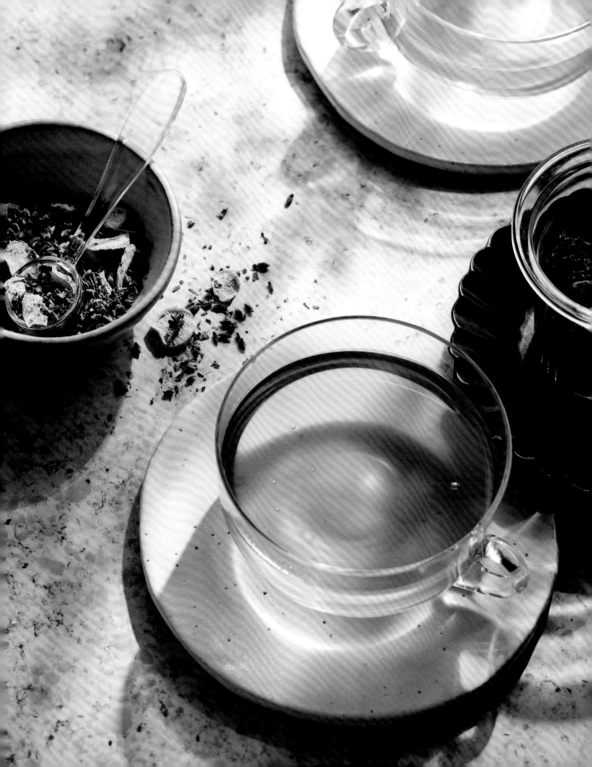

Dried Ginger Slices

Though more of the beneficial compounds are retained when ginger is dried in a microwave, drying it in a food dehydrator makes a more attractive finished product. Avoid drying ginger in the sun, which takes a couple of days, or in the oven, which can take many hours, because exposure to heat and air will degrade the nourishing components of herbs.

1 pound fresh ginger

MAKES ABOUT 1 CUP

• Start with plump, heavy ginger rhizomes with smooth skin (not wrinkled or moldy). Wash the ginger and pat dry.

• If the skin is young and smooth, you should be able to cleanly snap off the small fingers of ginger and you won't need to peel away the skin. If the ginger is older and more fibrous, cut away the small fingers with a knife, and remove the skin with a vegetable peeler or scrape it off with a knife.

• With a slicer or sharp knife, cut the ginger into very thin slices, no thicker than 1/8 inch. Uniform thickness allows them to dry evenly. You should have 3 to 4 cups of sliced ginger.

• To dry ginger in a food dehydrator, spread the slices on the trays, leaving space between the slices for air circulation. Dry at about 130 degrees F for 1 to 4 hours, until all moisture has evaporated.

• To dry ginger in a microwave, spread the slices on the clean glass turntable. In a standard 600-watt microwave at 100 percent power, cook for 30 seconds. Check for dryness. Remove any dry pieces, and flip the other pieces for uniform drying. Cook in additional 15-second intervals as needed. Watch closely to avoid browning and overcooking.

• Store fully dried ginger in an airtight container in a cool, dark place for up to 6 months.

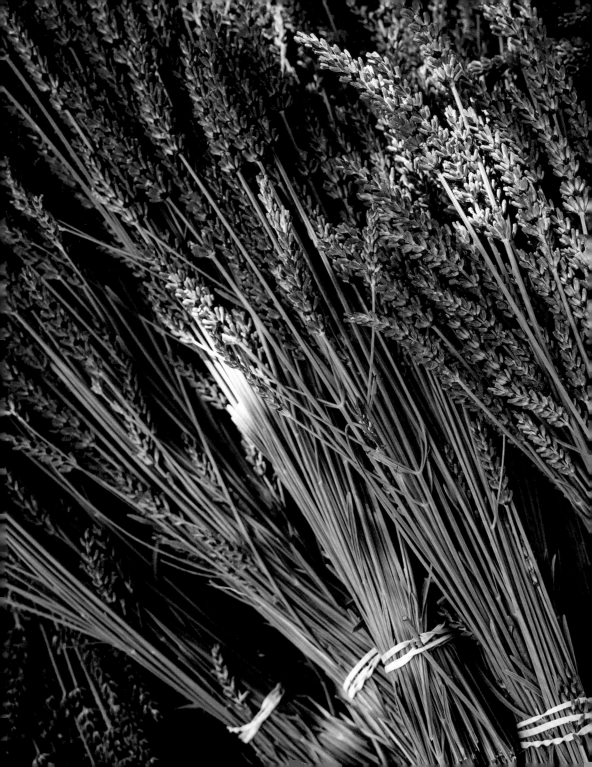

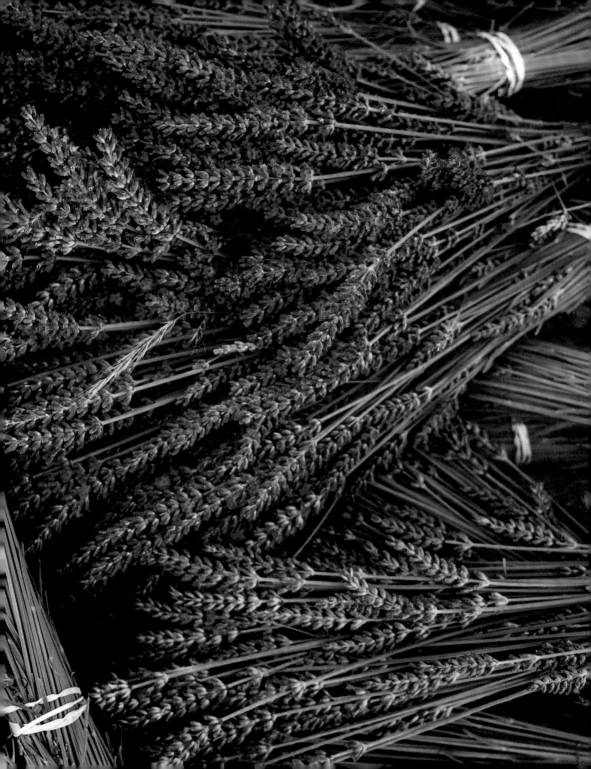

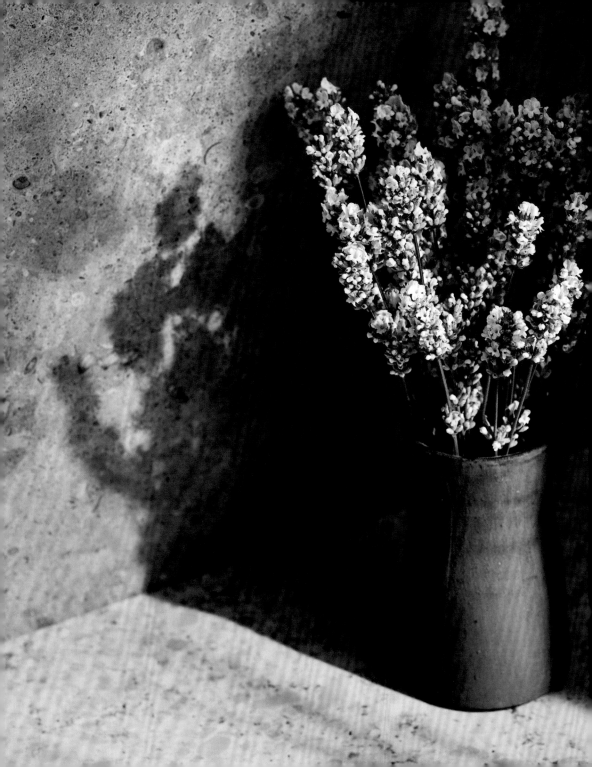

Special Thanks

For nearly every page here I could write about someone who has generously shared their expertise, time, ideas, lavender farm, or some other essential ingredient of this book. But then there'd be about 200 pages of acknowledgments and 1 page of lavender. So in this condensed and completely inadequate version, my humble thanks go to:

The whole Sasquatch team, and especially my editors: Hannah, for smoothing and shaping the good parts and whittling away the rest. You're a terrific editor, and equally an artist. And Rachelle, for guiding this book with all of its complexities to completion, all while under lockdown with three active complexities of your own.

My daughter and writing critique partner, Jill. Thanks for listening, reading, and always telling me—spot-on—what I need to hear.

My husband, Keith, for bravely tasting lavender recipes and never once complaining when the entire house was strewn with lavender projects and smelled like a purple field.

Victorie Inc., aromatherapy coach, for gently teaching me and being so patient with my never-ending essential oil questions. And Mesha, for teaching me to distill essential oil and letting me photograph butterflies flitting about your lavender field.

Dr. Desha Wood, for so carefully reviewing my essential oil research for safety. And Zion Hilliker, for reviewing and contributing those gems of hard-earned expertise on how to grow lavender.

A very special thanks to the farms whose lovely lavender plants and fields appear in this book:

- B & B Family Farm
- Fleurish Lavender of Lost Mountain
- Graysmarsh Farm
- Jardin du Soleil
- Kitty B's Lavender
- Lavender Connection
- Meshaz Lavender Farm
- Olympic Lavender Company
- Purple Haze Lavender Farm
- Victor's Lavender
- Victor's Rain Shadow Lavender
- Washington Lavender Farm

Michele and Gene, for recipe wisdom and for that fabulous lavender cocktail.

Cindy, for sharing your master gardening and lavender-crafting skills.

Sergei and Monica (Meli's Lavender), for teaching me to make a lavender wreath, and Mikey (Full Moon Candle Co.), for sharing candle-making tips.

Roger Mosley and Sally Harris, for sharing your photography expertise, and for helping my photos shine.

Lydia (traveling innkeeper and chef) and Kasydy and Dave (Let's Do Lavender), for generously testing so many recipes and crafts.

Catherine, the Herb Lady (Herbs 2 U Edible Landscaping), for sharing firsthand tips on how to successfully grow lavender in the scorching Arizona desert valley.

And finally the amazing lavender growers of Sequim who let me roam free on your farms to gather lavender flowers and pictures and answers—Bruce and Bonnie, Kristy and Zion, Susan and Doug, Victor and Maribel, Jeanette and Erich, Rick and Susan, Janet and Dan, Marco and Christa, Paul and Jordan, Amy and Jeff, Rex and Mary, and Mike. You've inspired me in a way that words never could, and I would not have written this book without you.

Resources

LAVENDER FARMS

Because I live in Sequim, Washington, which is often called America's Provence for its magnificent cluster of lavender farms and perfect lavender-growing climate, I'm naturally partial to our lavender growers and producers. Without reservation I can recommend any of their on-site and online offerings. Individual farms can be found at these websites:

SequimLavender.org

LavenderFestival.com/farms-in-our-association

LAVENDER PLANTS & TOOLS

PLANTS. When possible, buy plants from a local lavender farm or plant nursery that grows healthy lavender on-site. If ordering online, shorter shipping distances minimize stress on plants. These online sellers carry a good selection of lavender plants:

VictorsLavender.com (West Coast)

TheGrowers-Exchange.com (East Coast)

HighCountryGardens.com (South/Southwest)

HARVESTING SCYTHE. If you can't find a serrated sickle locally, you can find one online here:

AgricultureSolutions.com

RECIPE & PROJECT SUPPLIES

LAVENDER BUDS AND BUNDLES. Buy fresh and dried lavender from a lavender farm in your area, if available. For online purchases of quality dried *L. angustifolia* or lavandin, this farm store is tops:

BBFamilyFarm.com/shop

ESSENTIAL OILS, HYDROSOLS, CARRIER OILS, AND BOTANICALS. Mountain Rose Herbs is a favorite source for organic, ethically sourced, purity guaranteed, batch-tested essential oils. All their oils include a "packed on" date to ensure freshness. You'll also find vanilla absolute, quality carrier oils, vitamin E oil, aloe vera gel, rainbow peppercorns, brown mustard seeds, dried ginger, and dried botanicals, including rose petals, lemon balm, chamomile, peppermint, and calendula in their online shop:

MountainRoseHerbs.com

BOTTLING AND BLENDING SUPPLIES AND INGREDIENTS. For tools like tins, spray bottles, tubes, and inhalers, along with specialty ingredients such as Natrasorb Bath, witch hazel, arrowroot powder, butters, and citric acid, you'll find a good selection here:

AromaTools.com

DIFFUSERS. For a lovely selection of quality diffusers, try this website:

Asakuki.com

CANDLE- AND SOAP-MAKING SUPPLIES. This shop carries products such as coconut wax, thermometers, and wicks; you can also find copper stills for essential oil distillation:

CandlesandSupplies.net

UNSCENTED BASES. For making personal products, you can find a wide selection of unscented bases at this popular website:

BulkApothecary.com/unscented-bases

BEESWAX AND HONEY. This cruelty-free, bee-loving company offers small and bulk quantities of honey and beeswax produced by Florida and South Dakota bees:

BeeswaxfromBeekeepers.com

BOOKS

Essential Oil Safety by Robert Tisserand (seek out the most recent edition)

Essential Oils: A Comprehensive Handbook for Aromatic Therapy by Jennifer Peace Rhind

Candle Making Basics by Eric Ebeling

ONLINE ARTICLES

For extensive and well-researched aromatherapy and essential oil information:

AromaWeb.com

For safety, essential oil training, and reliable information:

TisserandInstitute.org/blog

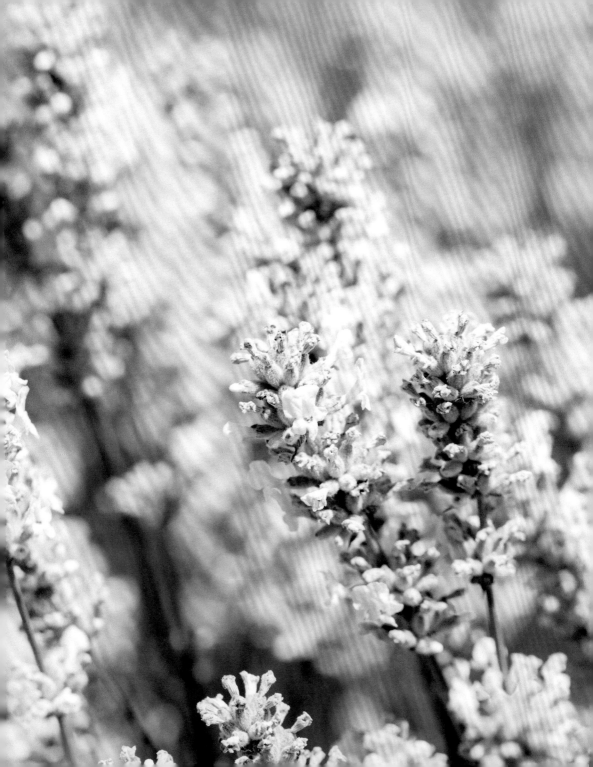

A Note on Sources

To access the books and scientific articles from which I gathered lavender research, you can download the endnotes and bibliography from:

http://bit.ly/SasquatchBooksLavenderBibliography

The numbered references in that document match the superscripted notations within this book.

Index

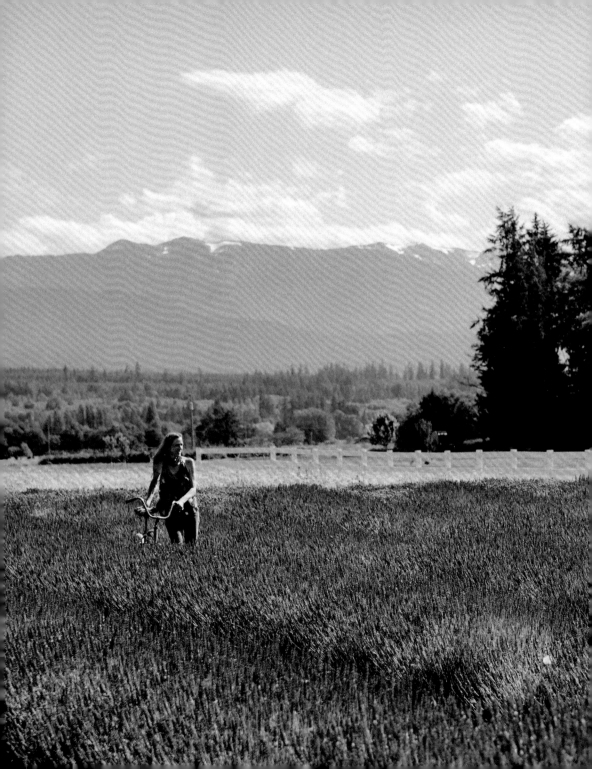

About the Author

BONNIE LOUISE GILLIS is the author/editor of 28 gift books, many of which were published under Bonnie Louise Kuchler. She lives surrounded by the lavender farms of Sequim, Washington, a place where mountains touch the sea and ancient trees breathe. Her favorite neighbors are a family of black-tailed deer, and her biggest thoughts come from tiny sprouts and towering evergreens.

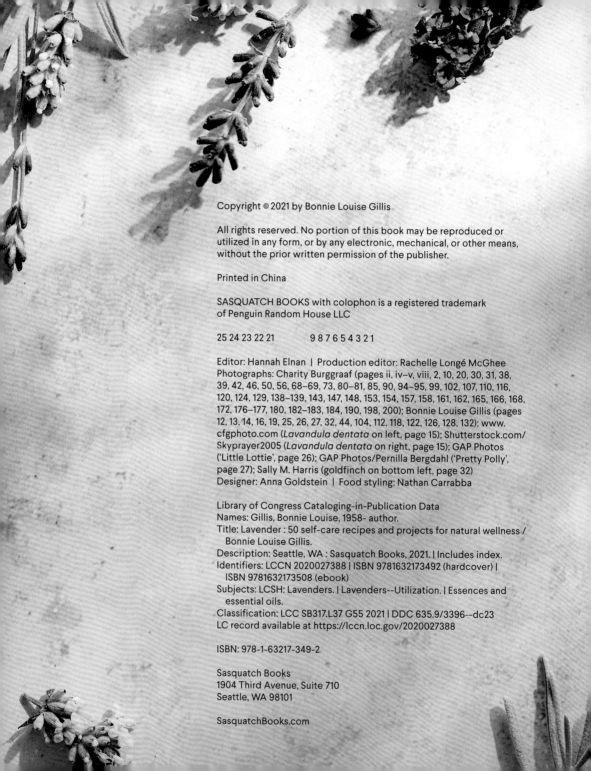

Printed in China

SASQUATCH BOOKS with colophon is a registered trademark of Penguin Random House LLC

25 24 23 22 21   9 8 7 6 5 4 3 2 1

Editor: Hannah Elnan | Production editor: Rachelle Longé McGhee
Photographs: Charity Burggraaf (pages ii, iv–v, viii, 2, 10, 20, 30, 31, 38, 39, 42, 46, 50, 56, 68–69, 73, 80–81, 85, 90, 94–95, 99, 102, 107, 110, 116, 120, 124, 129, 138–139, 143, 147, 148, 153, 154, 157, 158, 161, 162, 165, 166, 168, 172, 176–177, 180, 182–183, 184, 190, 198, 200); Bonnie Louise Gillis (pages 12, 13, 14, 16, 19, 25, 26, 27, 32, 44, 104, 112, 118, 122, 126, 128, 132); www.cfgphoto.com (*Lavandula dentata* on left, page 15); Shutterstock.com/Skyprayer2005 (*Lavandula dentata* on right, page 15); GAP Photos ('Little Lottie', page 26); GAP Photos/Pernilla Bergdahl ('Pretty Polly', page 27); Sally M. Harris (goldfinch on bottom left, page 32)
Designer: Anna Goldstein | Food styling: Nathan Carrabba

Library of Congress Cataloging-in-Publication Data
Names: Gillis, Bonnie Louise, 1958- author.
Title: Lavender : 50 self-care recipes and projects for natural wellness / Bonnie Louise Gillis.
Description: Seattle, WA : Sasquatch Books, 2021. | Includes index.
Identifiers: LCCN 2020027388 | ISBN 9781632173492 (hardcover) | ISBN 9781632173508 (ebook)
Subjects: LCSH: Lavenders. | Lavenders--Utilization. | Essences and essential oils.
Classification: LCC SB317.L37 G55 2021 | DDC 635.9/3396--dc23
LC record available at https://lccn.loc.gov/2020027388

ISBN: 978-1-63217-349-2

Sasquatch Books
1904 Third Avenue, Suite 710
Seattle, WA 98101

SasquatchBooks.com